What Others Are Saying About This

"I used to buy perfume because it smelled good or a girlfriend, or because a salesclerk recommended it to me as *the one everyone is buying*. [...] *Looking Hot and Loving Yourself,* I know how to te[...] body chemistry or not, as well as why I shouldn't car[...] know what sort of scent to wear if I'm on a date or [...] indoors, or outdoors."

—Misty Denton, 17

"One of the many wonderful features of this book is that it helps teens feel as though they are not alone in facing the tumultuous time of adolescence. Jennifer has certainly built a case for the glow that only knowing and understanding yourself can illuminate and has given teens the tools to 'buff up' the inside, as well as the outside. Warm, witty, and welcome advice from a writer who knows how to get the message across to teenagers in language they can understand and appreciate. Teens will love *Feeling Great, Looking Hot and Loving Yourself!* It's a book I would have loved to have when I was a teen!"

—Suzee Vlk, J.D.
author, *The SAT I for Dummies, The ACT for Dummies*

"I've always hated to exercise. I even skipped P.E. classes as often as I could. What I learned in this book is that there's a difference between exercise and fitness, and that having a fit and toned body doesn't have to be misery and drudgery: You can get fit doing something as fun as Salsaerobics—which is great news because I *love* to dance! And I'm *definitely* telling my school about the New P.E."

—Emily Richie, 17

"*Feeling Great, Looking Hot and Loving Yourself* is an impressive life-skills manual for teens, helping them make the most of looking and feeling attractive, inside and out, so they have the confidence to be themselves. This is a real edge: The teen who likes the way she looks and feels is less likely to compromise her values in gaining acceptance from others. A must for every teenager!"

—Cathy Schmachtenberger
Books Are Fun

"Looking hot at my school is really important, so I'm always experimenting to get it right. But it seemed to me that all the other girls knew things that I didn't, tricks that always made them look great, leaving me feeling I was never going to get the hang of it—never having a 'look' of my own, never really knowing what to wear or how to wear it. After reading this book, I know how to be as cool as Tara Wellington, the cheerleader who sits across from me in English!"

—Destiny Radosevic, 16

"*Feeling Great, Looking Hot and Loving Yourself* covers just about every facet of beauty a teenage girl could be interested in—from hairstyles to clothes, colors to perfumes, makeups to manicures, fitting in to being 'in,' diet to exercise. Fun, informative and practical, it's the ultimate in health and beauty books for teens. Not only has Jennifer included an impressive section on inner beauty, she's also filled her book with real-life scenarios that teens can readily relate to, bringing topics to life. As the mother of three daughters, one of whom is still a teen, I strongly recommend this book for any young woman, age ten to twenty."

—Tina Moreno
youth drug- and substance-abuse counselor

"I never liked the way my body looked, but whenever I tried to diet, I got so tired and grouchy, I couldn't think straight. It wasn't worth it! Jennifer's book showed me I didn't need to lose weight at all—I'm the right weight for my bone structure. (What a relief!) I found out that wearing the right styles makes me look just great! Best of all, I'm no longer comparing myself to others. I'm feeling more comfortable in my own skin."

—Suzanne Reeves, 16

"I've been thinking about getting a tattoo and a tongue stud, so I was really interested in the section that addressed all the things I was wondering about. It even answered questions I would never have thought to ask."

—Sierra Farrel, 13

"I always thought I had low self-esteem. This book showed me that I didn't. I've decided to stop feeling bad about myself when someone drops me as their friend if I don't go along with everything they want me to, especially boyfriends. I've learned that when you believe in yourself, that can make you *appealing* to others. I love that idea. Trusting myself and believing in me makes me a beautiful person to be around. That's the best news I've come across all year!"

—Crystal Adams, 14

"As Jennifer says, 'You can't always change the things that make you look stressed, but you can change the way you react to them.' I like that idea, a lot!"

—Priscilla Dillon, 18

"When I read this book, what I really wanted it to tell me was how to look awesome in everything I wore, tricks to having gorgeous hair, and how to better do my makeup. And I did get a lot of really valuable information on all those topics, but what I loved the most was the reminder that beauty begins on the inside. Friends, faith, a sense of purpose and having clear goals are huge contributions to your beauty, too. This book is very reassuring to a girl's sense of self."

—Tanya Jamal, 16

"Traversing adolescence can be tricky, especially as it pertains to having confidence in one's appearance. This wonderful health and beauty guide can help teens understand that beauty is as much an inner quality as an outward one—and shows them how to attain both. Very informative, practical and easy to digest."

—Miriam Lodell
Michigan high-school educator

Feeling Great, Looking Hot & Loving Yourself!

Health, Fitness & Beauty for Teens

Jennifer Leigh Youngs

coauthor of *Taste Berries for Teens* and *Taste Berries for Teens Journal*

Foreword by **Bettie B. Youngs, Ph.D.**

coauthor of *Taste Berries for Teens* and *Taste Berries for Teens Journal*

Health Communications, Inc.
Deerfield Beach, Florida

www.hci-online.com

Library of Congress Cataloging-in-Publication Data

Youngs, Jennifer Leigh, date.
    Feeling great, looking hot & loving yourself! : health, fitness & beauty for teens / Jennifer Leigh Youngs; foreword by Bettie B. Youngs.
       p.   cm.
    Includes bibliographical references.
    ISBN 1-55874-767-2 (trade paper)
    1. Teenage girls—Health and hygiene—Juvenile literature. 2. Beauty, Personal, in children—Juvenile literature. 3. Physical fitness in youth—Juvenile literature. 4. Body image in adolescence—Juvenile literature. I. Title

RA777.25.Y68 2000
613.7'043—dc21
                                             99-088437

©2000 Jennifer Leigh Youngs and Bettie B. Youngs
ISBN 1-55874-767-2

Publisher: Health Communications, Inc.
             3201 S.W. 15th Street
             Deerfield Beach, FL 33442-8190

Cover design and inside illustrations by Lisa Camp
Inside book design and typesetting by Lawna Patterson Oldfield
Jennifer Leigh Youngs's computer-generated hairstyles in colorplates 57–71 and on page 296 by Susan Gilbert of New Looks on Video
Other hairstyles by Raymond David Farmer and Michele Heppner
Carrie Hague's before-and-after makeover by Lois Pearl
Other makeup and skin care by Sherie Darr, Karina Pawlukiewicz and Eva Szwaja
Professional photographs by Marty Mann
Scarves in colorplates 40–45 by Frankie Welch of Frankie Welch Designs

This book is dedicated with love to the three most beautiful women I've ever known:

To my mother, Bettie B. Youngs, an awesome presence with courage, radiance and grace. More than anyone else, it was she who taught me that life shrinks or expands in proportion to one's courage. Because of her, I *know* how beauty *manifests*. It is with this passionate woman with an undeniably mother's heart that I've experienced the blessings, honor and skill behind Anaïs Nin's words: "We write to taste life twice."

To my grandmother, Arlene Burres, who held my heart in the palm of her hand as we went for nature walks. It was on these many trips that she showed me the *truth* of beauty—from the intricacies of Mother Nature to the majestic door to God. It is from this wise woman that I have most learned the benevolence of C. G. Jung's words: "Who looks outside dreams; who looks inside wakes."

To a most lovely and gentle soul in the universe, Laurie Faye Burres, whose delicate and serene nature is evident in everything she does and in all the ways she does them. I get joyful even *thinking* about the fun and friendship we share. Her timeless devotion surely is what James Thurber referred to in his words, "*Love* is what you've been through with somebody."

Also by Jennifer Leigh Youngs:

Taste Berries for Teens: Inspirational Short Stories and Encouragement on Life, Love, Friendship and Tough Issues

Taste Berries for Teens Journal: My Thoughts on Life, Love and Making a Difference

Goal Setting Skills for Young Adults

A Stress Management Guide for Teens

Coming in September 2000:

MORE Taste Berries for Teens: Inspirational Short Stories and Encouragement on Life, Love, Friendship and Tough Issues

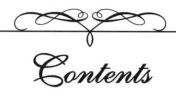

Contents

PART ONE: *Health & Beauty: From the Inside Out*

Food, Now!"—And Those Other All-Day-Long Cravings • A Recipe for Energy Bars You'll Love • Essential Vitamins and Minerals: What They Are and How to Make Sure You're Getting All You Need

Pizza or Soup?—How to Decide Which Is More Nutritious • Everything You Need to Know About Calories • How to Read a Food Label • Putting Chocolate-Dipped Potato Chips to the Test • Why Skipping Meals Is a Bad Idea • The Trick to Quieting a Screaming Taste Bud • Making Smart Choices About Food

What Should *You* Weigh? • Five Smart Ways to Watch Your Weight • Making Tasty Low-Calorie Foods—Great Recipes You'll Want to Try • Burning Calories by Exercising • How to Fight Cellulite • What You Should Know About Diet Pills—And Smoking

The Billion Benefits of "Buffing Up" • Becoming Your Own Xena the Warrior • An "A" for the Day—And for Life: Fifteen Minutes in Your Zone • Are You Getting Enough Exercise?—Rating Workout Activities • Getting Fit with Friends: Team Sports, Power Walking, "Challenge Exercise," Stretch Workouts, Dancing and Other Ways to "Buff Up" • Making Healthy Choices—Saying "No" to Things That Harm Your Body

22. Simply *Beautiful* Hair 285

Mane Advice: Seven Important Beauty Treatments for Having Beautiful Hair • How to Know What Shampoo Is Best for You • Should You Use a Creme Rinse or a Conditioner?—How to Tell • How to Choose a Hairstyle That's Right for You • Scissor Sizzle: Important Questions to Ask Your Stylist While Getting a Haircut • Highlighting and Coloring Your Hair • Wigs, Hair Extensions and Other Ways to Change Your Look

23. Dressing Up Your Face 305

Nine Steps to Creating a Beautiful Face • How to Choose the Right Makeup for You • Artful Applications: Great Ways with Eyeliner, Eyeshadow, Mascara, Blush, Concealer, Foundation and Lipstick • How to Change the Shape of Your Eyes • How to Have Great Eyebrows • A Before-and-After Makeover with Makeup Artist Lois Pearl

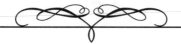

Acknowledgments

I would like to thank the many people who so generously offered their time and expertise in the development of this book. First, to all the teens with whom I've worked so closely over the past year who have contributed so much to this work, especially Carrie Hague, Kate MacIsaac, Lena Arcero, Renee Moreno, Talla Gowhari, Kelly Bull and Jenaye Quarles—a special taste-berry thanks; you are near and dear to my heart. To author Patricia Hill Burnett, designer Frankie Welch, photographer Marty Mann, self-care beauty experts Karina Pawlukiewicz, Lois Pearl, Ewa Szwaja, Sherie Darr and stylists Raymond David Farmer, Susan Gilbert and Michele Heppner. I honor your expertise and friendship.

To my publisher, Peter Vegso, at Health Communications—thanks for your belief and support of my work. And to Peter's talented staff, most especially the editorial department—Christine Belleris, Matthew Diener, Lisa Drucker, Allison Janse, Erica Orloff—your encouragement and professional assistance is just the *best!* And to graphic designer Lisa Camp, your work is, as teens would say, "way cool," and "very hot!" My mother is fond of saying that some of the most important roles in life are akin to housework: Nobody knows what you do unless you *don't* do it. So thanks to the many others at HCI for your important roles in sending this book into the world of readers. A huge thanks to Tina Moreno of our staff. While I'm flying across the country to do workshops and book signings, she's in the office keeping my projects grounded. Tina, I'm always grateful for your calm in the midst of the storm of my activity!

Deepest appreciation to my mother, Bettie B. Youngs, who gives me a sense of roots—of belonging—as well as wings to fly, professionally and in all areas of my life. She's my number-one fan and I love that. More than anyone else, it was she who taught me about beauty—from the inside, out—teaching me most by her example, clarity and her unfailing belief in my personal best. The best way to thank my mother is simply to hug her. We share a heart—and for me, it's a feeling of love and connection and support. And to my grandmother, Arlene Burres. This glorious woman is a pillar of strength to me and to every member of her family. I have boundless love for her. I also want to give thanks for the loyal and loving support of some my favorite "guys": My grandfather Everett Burres, a genuine caretaker and the best grandpa a girl could have; "Good-guy" Dic Youngs, my father, a most honorable man; David Kirk, who is never too tired or too short on time—and advice! And to the many friends who give me room to grow and support me as I do that. And to Timber and Kitty, my kitties, who sat at my feet or as close to the keyboard of my computer as they could get while I was writing. They need love and take love with surprising acuity to my needs and I adore them for it! And, as always, I give glory to God, from whom all blessings flow.

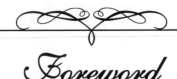

Foreword

Dear Teen Reader,

Being a teenager is an exciting—and confusing—time. You feel on top of the world one day, and down in the dumps the next. You feel self-confident one day, only be greeted by self-doubt the next. You look in the mirror and feel quite sure that you are positively looking like hot stuff and then, before you know it, your great-hair day, your radiant complexion and your good mood take a drastic U-turn. Who needs it?

Adolescence is like that. But no one needs to tell you about the pros and cons of being a teen. So instead, let me tell you a little about the author of this book. Her name is Jennifer Leigh Youngs and she is my daughter. When she was born, she looked and behaved like most babies: she was cute, had very wrinkled skin, scowled a lot, and her screaming for food terrified the family dog. I love her beyond words and have always wanted the best for her, but even so, she had to deal with life like everyone else: day-by-day.

She was a cute little girl, but by fourth grade was feeling "oblong and ugly." Having looked like Cinderella throughout much of her childhood, she wondered out loud how nature could have dealt her such a cruel blow. Now she was gangly and uncoordinated, her facial features were elongating and filling out—and not all at the same time. She was really upset about it. She complained and complained, and no reassurance on my part could appease her.

One day Jennifer and I were going through a box of old pictures and came across all my childhood pictures that my mother had kept for me. Jennifer was very interested in these old photos—one more so than the others. The particular photo that caught her attention was one of me with an extraordinarily goofy grin on my face, oversized front teeth and the two on either side of them missing. As she described it, I looked like the "Ultimate Geek." She flipped the photo over and there, in my mother's beautiful handwriting, was, "Bettie in fourth grade." My daughter rolled on the floor with laughter!

With a better understanding that a picture is worth a thousand words, I gathered up my childhood photos, arranged them in a year-by-year chronology, then had them put into one large frame. I hung this array of photos in the hallway outside her room. My daughter visited these photos quite often over the years, most especially when she was in her teens. I have no doubt that they helped her accept that with each year comes a new and different "look"—and perhaps helped her gain a little tolerance for all the changes she was going through, both physically and emotionally. At least I'd like to think so. One day when she was in the tenth grade, my daughter asked, "Mom, when you were a sophomore, did anyone ask you to the junior-senior prom?" I thought she was warming up to ask me if she could accept a date to go to the junior-senior prom. But, when I replied, "No, no such luck," she remarked, "It probably had something to do with how 'nerdy' you looked in that *phase!*" Then, upon reviewing an assortment of other photos of me during my high school years, Jennifer remarked, "Mom, you sure did change a lot from year to year. How is it possible to be so cool one year and nerdy the next?"

Adolescence is like that. So many changes, inside and out. Different looks, different feelings.

What Jennifer learned and wants you to understand is that much of what you see and how you feel during the teen years belongs to a "stage of development," albeit an intense one. But keep in mind that all of us, at every age in our lives, are in a constant process of changing. Most of us may like our appearance a great deal one year, and the next only so-so. Or, we may be quite happy with the results of one stage, and wish we could skip other changes altogether!

Maybe right now you are going through a great phase—one in which you are healthy and happy and feeling good about yourself. Maybe your body feels energized rather than lazy from all the growing and hormonal changes going on. If so, great! But if you aren't feeling quite like Cinderella at the ball, remember that it's just that, a phase. Just ask your parents; they know from experience. I'll bet they have some photos of themselves much like those Jennifer discovered of me—photos that showed them in various stages of looking hot, and in Jennifer's words for me in tenth grade, "nerdy." We all change, especially in the teen years. As Jason, one of Jennifer's friends, said to me, "I look totally different than I did just three months ago because then I had a decent complexion, and now it's oily and zit-ridden. Then I had a great physique; now my body parts look like they don't belong with the other parts. Now, from one day to the next, my emotions are all over the place. *Everything* is changing! I'm looking forward to the time when the real me will stay around long enough for me to get used to!"

For Jason, it may be awhile. He just turned fifteen! But even though adolescence is a time of many changes—and some of them, like extra-oily skin you'd like to do without—there are some things you can do to feel good and look great while your body is moving from this stage to the next. This practical health, fitness and beauty guide can help you look and feel attractive, inside and out, as you go through the tumultuous time of adolescence and help you answer questions that practically every teenager asks: What's with my ever-changing emotions and feelings? How can I understand them, much less cope? How can I look great all the time—even when I'm feeling so not "with it"? How can I feel self-confident and sure of myself when I'm not as attractive as others? How can I fit in, be one of the "cool" kids? What is the best way to care for my skin and hair, especially now that it's extra oily? How can I look great? What are the secrets of "cool"? What can I do to make the most of *my* looks, my body, my appearance?

These and a million other questions are asked by teens the world over. It's only natural to want to look and feel your best. There are practical benefits as well. Liking the way you look and feel can be a real edge in helping you be yourself around others. The more authentic you are—the more you stay true to the person you are—the less likely you will compromise yourself or your values to gain approval and acceptance from others. Having taught both junior and senior high school—not to mention having a house full of teenagers when my daughter was an adolescent—I have a better appreciation for the ups and downs teens go through in this incredible time of growth, and especially for how tough it can be to go through this stage *with other teens!* As teens compare themselves to their peers, they often judge each other harshly and can be cruel in their remarks to each other. The more you like and accept yourself, the more confident you will be keeping these comments in perspective; this can take the sting out of having your feelings hurt.

My daughter has blossomed out of her gangly phase and has become a lovely young woman. Like many of her classmates, she breezed through some phases, and grumbled and mumbled her way through others. Jennifer, now twenty-five, is a soulful person—one who sees people and life through the eyes of her heart. She has an eye for beauty, a nose for common sense and an extraordinarily large funny bone. She is a young woman who is comfortable in her own skin, and would love for you to be, too. Her advice in this book is simple: Value your health and do not sacrifice it. Believe in yourself and make friends with the face in the mirror. Have the courage to be an individual; be aware of others around you; be friendly and courteous, but don't forget that you are you. Appreciate yourself; learn to enjoy the feeling of being healthy, fit and attractive on your terms. Be as healthy, fit and beautiful as you can be—but never lose sight of the fact that *you* get to decide what that means for you. Offer up *your* brand of beauty; *you* are who the world is waiting to see and learn all about.

If you will take this advice, you will reach the same happy conclusion as Jennifer: With each year there is a growing sense of self-confidence in your own style and in your own individual beauty. While we live in a world filled with others, we are each one-of-a-kind. Love that person, and we will, too.

Taste Berries to you!
Bettie B. Youngs, Ph.D.

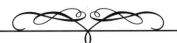

Introduction

One of the fun things about being a teenager today is that we have more options than ever: We can go from looking casual to looking glamorous, from looking sophisticated to looking outrageous, from fitting in to making a statement. We can wear our natural-color hair or wear it purple if we like. We can have straight hair one day, and kinky hair the next; short hair one day and then, with the magic of hair extensions, long hair the next day. With the wave of a wand we can change our brown eyes to blue eyes, or our blue eyes to green eyes. We have so many choices, so many options, so many "looks" to chose from; what fun!

Fashion and style isn't the only domain where there are oh so many options to define ourselves. While being in "shape" was once akin to how much you weighed, today "being in shape" means having a healthy body, one that is energized and can keep up with *you!* What's more, how we get and stay fit has been jazzed-up with exercise options ranging from aerobics to yoga, from sports to Salsaerobics. Keeping fit is not only important to your health, but it can be fun to achieve, too!

With so many possibilities—and "beautiful" and "fit" being redefined—doing a book on health, fitness and beauty was quite a challenge. Where to start? What to cover? What is most hip, cool, best, better, prettier, the most beautiful? Who is to say that wearing makeup is a more glamorous look than au natural? The answers are always personal: What is best for you is, well, what is best for *you*. It's a matter of personal taste—but try convincing yourself of that! "Best for you" is an underlying goal in this book. Consider this your personal guide to being your personal best, a guide to help you think about what's important to you in being your best, and then ways to be *your* best—inside and out.

There are a lot of ways to polish our own natural inner and outer beauty. Whether you want to add the inner radiance of self-confidence or purposeful goals, the outer glow of a complexion that shines with health, the luster of hair that gleams with vitality, the facet of fitness, or the magic of makeup—it's just a matter of your desire to achieve it.

This book is divided into four units:

Unit 1: The Essential Attributes of Beauty is all about the ways that beauty manifests from within. Have you ever run across someone who looked stunning, but undid her beauty by the way she acted or treated others? Compare that to someone who is thoughtful and has a kind heart, confident and comfortable with herself and as a result, has a lovely presence about her. What is the difference between lovely and beautiful? The difference is inner harmony—and it's a *huge* part of true beauty. This unit shows you how to let your inner beauty shine through—things like the secrets of serenity, steps for staying cool under pressure, building your self-esteem, drawing security from loving others, setting goals and feeling purposeful.

Unit 2: Health, Fitness & Nutrition covers a most essential topic for teens: having a healthy body, liking your body and being fit, or as teens say, "looking hot." This can be more difficult to achieve than you might imagine. In the teen years, our bodies (and moods) are in a constant state of change. We can feel like we're just getting to know who we are when suddenly we are someone totally different. While the ups and downs caused by all the hormonal changes going on can make you and your body feel like you are strangers to each other, it's most important that you be friends. This unit uncovers some of the myths teens have for comparing themselves to a standard other than their own, and covers some very important ground on how to best take care of your body so you look and feel *your* very best. Learn how to decide what weight is best for *you;* how to fuel your body and make smart choices when it comes to food, as well as important information on the subject of weight loss. And yes, the importance of buffing up those muscles—and relaxing them as well.

Do you find that you often buy clothes on impulse—because the item is trendy or the price is right—and then end up almost never wearing it because it just doesn't look quite right on you? If so, the really fun and fact-filled **Unit 3: Clothes, Colors & Accessories** will show you how to select clothes that look great on you, everything from what clothes look best on *your* body to why a certain color makes you feel and look better than do others, including advice on what jewelry looks best with what. Then there's my favorite chapter, Scents-ible Advice—one I'm sure you'll love, too—which explains why a perfume can smell good on you one season but not another, and how to choose the best scent for *you*. There's also a chapter filled with tips for being a smart shopper when you get to the mall!

Unit 4: Skin Care, Hair & Makeup Magic is about appeasing the Cinderella in all of us, granting all sorts of valuable advice on everything from how to have a beautiful complexion and gorgeous hair, to how to have attractive nails, hands and feet. Step-by-step, you'll learn how to work makeup magic—tricks with foundation, mascara, eye shadow, eye liner, lipstick, lipliner and more!

So much information, so many suggestions; still, it was impossible to cover everything, a fact that really comes clear in consulting with "beauty experts" out there. (Be sure to check out the suggested reading section at the end of this book!) One thing the experts did agree on: When it comes to how you look and how you feel—your health and beauty—you are the most important "expert" of all. So, do what works for *you,* work on what feels right to *you,* experiment with new techniques, have fun and—most important—remember that we each carry our greatest source of health and beauty within. Decide to value this, and make your personal best the standard for you! So here's to your feeling great, looking hot, and loving yourself—inside and out!

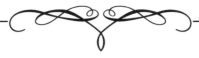

PART ONE

Health & Beauty: From the Inside Out

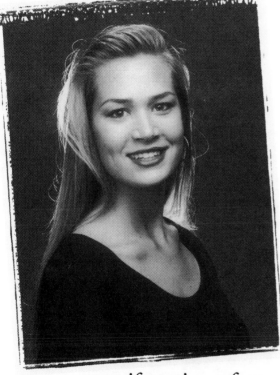

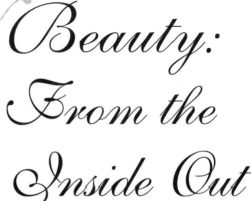

Everything that occurs—everything that has occurred —is occurring, and ever will occur—is the outward physical manifestation of your innermost thoughts, choices, ideas and determination regarding Who You Are and Who You Choose to Be.

—God, in Neale Donald Walsch's *Conversations with God,* Book 3

The Essential Attributes of Beauty

The work of life is to grow closer to who we really are, closer to the image of the person we know to be ourselves.

—Taste Berries for Teens

Inventory:
For Sale! Inner Beauty Galore!

You know how important it is to have all the right things to look hot and feel good—things like trendy clothes and jewelry, the very latest in beauty products, such as the newest in lip gloss, perfume and nail colors. Shopping, shopping, constantly shopping—it's a lot of fun to keep up with fads, fashions and trends. But there are some things that money just can't buy—things like love, self-esteem, faith, friends and goals that give your life real purpose. Yet, these priceless and precious qualities can make a girl more appealing and attractive than any of the latest or most expensive store purchases—and their worth goes far beyond anything that all the money in the world can buy. See for yourself. If you could have any ten of the following "attributes," which would you chose?

- ❑ Having all the confidence in the world
- ❑ Having a real sense of purpose
- ❑ Success at everything I do
- ❑ Knowing what I want out of life
- ❑ Having others (especially my parents) always believe in me
- ❑ Liking everything about my life
- ❑ Having many good friends
- ❑ Being genuinely happy and content
- ❑ Being considered a sensational girlfriend
- ❑ Having "grace under pressure" so I never lose my cool
- ❑ Being the most popular girl at my school
- ❑ Perspective—knowing *now* all those things people are referring to when they say, "I wish I knew then what I know now"
- ❑ Having healthy self-esteem
- ❑ Being part of a family where everyone loves each other and gets along
- ❑ Feeling really sure of myself
- ❑ Compassion for others
- ❑ Loving myself—being patient with me and forgiving myself when I mess up
- ❑ Being a good and great citizen of the world
- ❑ Knowing that I'm always true to what I truly believe

❑ Caring deeply about every living being (and creature) in the world

❑ Being liked by everybody

❑ Being able to "act" beautiful, even when I'm not feeling that way

❑ Having absolute faith in a Higher Power

❑ Being the person who comes up with the solution for world hunger

❑ Having peace of mind

❑ Never getting stressed out

❑ Being a possibility thinker, so I always think positive

❑ Having a lifetime guarantee of never being dependent on alcohol or other drugs

Now look back over your list and rank the ten you selected in their order of importance or value to you (1 being the most important and 10 being the least).

Was it tough to decide on only ten? As a teenager, it's sometimes difficult to know exactly what you want, especially when you're still just learning about yourself. It helps if you think about what's really important in life—what matters most—and then develop the inner courage to "go for it." This unit will show you how.

1

If Only I Had Known in High School What I Know Now!

Life is a challenge—Meet it!
Life is a song—Sing it!
Life is a dream—Realize it!
Life is a game—Play it!
Life is love—Enjoy it!

—Sri Sathya Sai Baba

Beauty Begins on the Inside

One of the things I liked best—and least—about being a teenager was the excitement of things being so "do or die!" For me, every little thing—every single word, action and even the thoughts of my family and friends (of course I always *just knew* what they were thinking)—was crucial, urgent and dire. For example, when I was in high school, if I wanted to go out with a certain guy, I hoped, planned and prayed that he would ask me out. I worried one minute that he wouldn't ask and worried the next minute what I would do or say if and when he did. Then, when the guy did ask me out, I fretted that I

7

somehow wouldn't measure up to his previous girlfriend—who I always pictured as drop-dead gorgeous, popular with everyone with whom she came into contact, brilliant and talented, and with a great body that was buffed to the max. Never mind that I didn't know her, nor had I ever even seen her. Never mind that I was a good athlete, was often on the honor roll and had many good friends. Somehow, I never really figured out that I could compete on my own merits. I worried about everything. Everything was such a big deal.

The Ultimate "Drama-Mama"

As agonizing as all this was, I didn't let it interfere with my being even more of a "drama-mama." On the day of the big date, I would be simply devastated if my hair wasn't exactly perfect, if my complexion wasn't as clear as I hoped it would be; or if I didn't feel that I looked *exactly* as spectacular as I wanted. Then, even though my date and I had a nice time on that first date, I next worried about whether or not my heartthrob would ask me out *again*. When he did, I wondered if—and when—we would have date three, four, and five. You get the idea.

When the boyfriend became "my guy," *getting-a-guy anxiety* gave way to *keeping-my-guy anxiety*. Now the task in my head was to make sure everyone knew Romeo and I were a "solid" couple, that our soul-mate-love-made-in-heaven was *forever,* so they better "stay off my turf."

Of course, the guy was probably going through a similar charade as well, one complete with its own doubts and insecurities. But I didn't let that limit me from having fears of my own. The more the merrier!

So whether it was guys, grades, good friends or the way I looked and dressed, I put myself through the paces. *Everything* was "do or die."

Brad Wilson: "To Die For"

Today at twenty-five, I still have a life filled with complex and anxiety-ridden situations, only now things no longer seem so "do or die!" Experience has taught me to take things in stride and to trust myself more. And this trust makes all the difference in the world. For example, six months ago I met a great-looking guy (Brad Wilson) who asked me out for the following Saturday night. We agreed he'd pick me up at seven o'clock.

I was really looking forward to going out with Brad. On each of the several occasions I'd talked with him prior to his asking me out, I found him to be stylish, smart and savvy, funny, and as we would say in high school, "cool" and "to die for." So when *the* Saturday arrived, I bounded out of bed and headed for work in a better mood than usual (I work every other Saturday from 10:00 to 5:00). I was really looking forward to the evening. The day flew by!

Because I was off work at five o'clock, I knew I'd have ample time to run the two errands I needed to get done: picking up my hot new blazer and skirt from the cleaners so I could wear them on my date with Brad, and stopping at the city library to pick up a research book for an important college term paper due the following Monday. My brain had a time schedule all worked out: off at 5:00, to the cleaners by 5:15, at the library at 5:30, home by 6:00. Once at home, I'd do a quick twenty-minute pick-me-up workout with my favorite workout video to reenergize, then put on my favorite CD, take a relaxing bubble bath and have thirty minutes to dress for my big date!

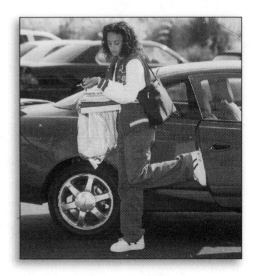

Regardless of my being organized, things didn't go as planned! It fact, it took only ten minutes for things to begin to unravel! The employee who takes over when I leave at 5:00 called in sick. I found this out when the store manager phoned me and asked if I would please stay until he came in to cover for the sick employee. Of course, I said I would.

The manager said he would be at the store in twenty minutes—only he didn't arrive until 5:50!

Getting off work at 5:50 instead of 5:00 really cut into the time I'd planned for the leisurely and relaxed evening before my date arrived. Nevertheless, I left work the instant my manager arrived and headed straight for the cleaners, only to discover that the cleaners had already closed for the day. Although this was upsetting, I headed immediately to the library. I couldn't skip this errand because the city library is closed on Sundays, so I had no option but to go check out the book I needed for the paper I'd planned to do the next day. At least I thought I'd be checking out the book. When I got to the library, I found that the book hadn't been returned!

In short, not only were things not going as planned, but I was running very late. So late that I arrived home only minutes before my "to die for" date arrived!

Grace Under Pressure

If something similar had happened to me as a teenager, I would have been beside myself, working myself into a frenzy. Then I would have been in a bad mood, and who knows what kind of an evening I would have created. But now I'm learning to relax a bit, to take things in stride, and to work with each situation—especially those that require grace under pressure. So when Brad knocked at the door, I opened it and said politely, "It's wonderful to see you. I'm running about twenty minutes late. Come in and make yourself comfortable. If we need to reschedule dinner reservations, the phone is in the kitchen. I'll tell you all about it over dinner!"

Then, twenty minutes later, Brad and I left my apartment and went to dinner. My hair was not having the best of days, and I was not wearing the hot new blazer and skirt that I had hoped to wear. Even so, I made the best of it and selected my next-favorite outfit. As upsetting as it was that the research book I had planned on using for my term paper had not been returned to the library like it was supposed to have been, I decided I'd have to figure out a contingency plan the next day. I didn't have the benefit of reenergizing after a long day at work, or the benefit of relaxation time so as to switch gears from the "mental briefcase" of work-related problems. And the much-desired bubble bath where I had intended to dreamily anticipate the evening with Brad . . . well, that went down the drain (!) as well.

From "Ghoul" to "Cool"

I've learned that when things don't go as planned, when they aren't exactly the way you'd like them to be, you have to make the best of what you have. When

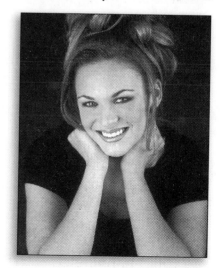

you're stressed out or worrying about every little thing, it takes away from your "cool"—from looking and acting "together." With my new date, I simply had to get comfortable with the fact that I'd had a particularly hectic day and make the decision that I wasn't going to drag it along with me to dinner with Brad.

If only I had known in high school what I know now, I could have saved myself a lot of undue stress and looked a lot more cool to boot.

The secret of getting from A to B—from drama-mama to cool—is this: You can't always control the outer world, but you can control how you respond—how you act—in relation to what's going on around you. Unlike those things that you have little say or control over, such as the natural color of your eyes or an occasional bad hair day, the qualities that radiate your cool *are* under your control. Those qualities include a positive attitude and a decision to remain calm and focus on the solutions, rather than the problems at hand. [Check out the suggested reading section at the back of this book for ways to manage stress.] Just as you put on an outfit that looks hot on you, or wear your hair in a style that compliments your face, or wear fingernail polish, lipstick or mascara to add color and pizzazz, you can greatly enhance the color of your cool. It's a *choice* you make to draw control from within. This choice becomes visible in a poised beauty that shines through you.

A Secret of Inner Beauty: "Act" Beautiful

You carry your beauty with you every minute of every day, every place you go. I'll never forget the evening when a small group of us were returning from touring several of the old Southern plantations in Charleston, South Carolina, where we were attending Renaissance Weekend. A four-day event, Renaissance days began bright and early at seven o'clock. After the plantation tours, we went to dinner. After a ten-hour conference, then touring and dinner, I don't mind telling you, I was dragging!

It was nearly 11:30 at night, and I was slouched in the small transport van in the seat beside eighty-year-old Patricia Hill Burnett [see page 51 and colorplate 39]. Exhausted and bleary-eyed, I gazed over at Patricia, sitting perfectly erect.

Her chin up, she looked poised and lovely, every bit like a grand Southern belle. "Aren't you tired?" I inquired, puzzled by her apparently endless energy and the fact that she could still look so composed, refreshed and beautiful after the day we'd had. "I'm exhausted," I said, "and quite sure I look it. But you look so fresh and perky, as though you've napped. Have you?"

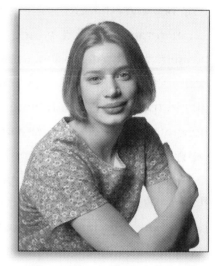

"Oh, no," she replied, admitting, "It's been quite a long day and I am most definitely tired."

"But you look so radiant, so beautiful," I remarked. "I've used up my allotment for the day. *How do you do it?*"

With her customary warmth and tenderness, Patricia reached for my hand, looked me in the eyes, and in her style of speaking while at the same time smiling, pointed to her head and said sweetly, "I keep a little reserve of beauty right up here." Laughing softly, she added, "You are only as beautiful as you feel *on the inside*. Beauty is from the inside out. And, just as they say about sunshine, you have to carry it with you! To be beautiful, you must act beautiful."

Patricia's radiance comes not only from being beautiful, but also from *acting* beautiful. It's one of the great secrets of beauty: Beauty comes from within.

It is primarily from this vantage point—beauty from the inside out—that we are beautiful.

Like Money in the Bank: The Glow of Inner Beauty

Inner beauty has a powerful glow, one that is clearly visible to those around you. Perhaps you know someone like my friend, Patricia, whose inner beauty shines so brightly you describe her as "a beautiful person." Unfortunately, some people are beautiful outside . . . and not so pretty inside. Perhaps you know someone who possesses great physical beauty but whose lack of inner vibrancy overshadows or even cancels out her outer beauty.

I'm reminded of a young man who wrote telling me he'd met a girl he thought was the "most beautiful girl he had ever seen." Finally he got up the courage to ask her out. When she accepted, he thought he was the luckiest guy in the world. The feeling was short-lived. As he began to get to know her, he saw a person who was very different from what he had imagined. He discovered the girl wasn't very kind and respectful of other people, qualities he associated with her not being happy within herself. After dating her for only five weeks, the young man decided not to ask the girl out anymore. "Seeing her beauty, I thought she must *be* beautiful," he wrote, "but as I got to see the real person, I could tell that her beauty was all on the outside, just an outward appearance. Even that wasn't lasting: When she didn't have her makeup on, she didn't think she was pretty and it showed in the way she treated others. I've learned that if a person doesn't feel pretty on the inside, then even though she is beautiful to look at, the advantage is shallow. When inner beauty is missing, your feelings of attraction for that person wear off. Being pretty on the outside can only get you so far."

So how do you acquire inner beauty? It's not elusive. As this unit will show you, acquiring inner beauty is largely about:

- Drawing inspiration from the sources that tie us to timeless truths.
- Developing a positive sense of self.
- Interacting with others in positive ways.
- Knowing what you want out of life and having purposeful goals.
- Managing your response to stress.

• Caring for yourself by keeping yourself healthy and fit.

So how did things turn out with my "to die for" date? Great! At the end of a really nice evening, I said simply, "Thank you for being so patient with me this evening." My date was impressed with my "cool"—and so was I.

And seven months later, I'm still dating Brad!

2

The Radiance of Inner Beauty

*People are like stained glass windows.
They sparkle and shine when the sun is out; but
when the darkness sets in their true beauty is
revealed only if there is a light inside.*

—ELISABETH KÜBLER-ROSS

Nature—Good for Your Heart and Soul

I love to go bike riding with my friends because biking is good exercise and a great way to spend time with them. But another reason is that being outdoors, being in the midst of nature is good for my heart and soul. Nature can help us get in touch with the bigger world we live in.

Picture that you and several of your best friends have ridden your bikes to the top of a steep hill, where you stop to rest. You look into a vast blue horizon where clouds that look like tufts of cotton balls lounge like lazy alligators sunning on a river bank on a hot summer's day. You look down into an immense valley of lush green trees and hearty ground-shrubs sprinkled with patches of wildflowers, a picturesque landscape—a sharp contrast to the teeny-tiny flowers decorating the ground beneath your feet.

You are filled with an appreciation for the wonder and beauty of nature, one that leaves you with a feeling of awe and serenity.

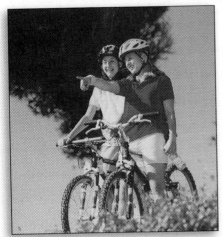

As though she notices your appreciation—perhaps by your tranquil smile or from the lengthy breath of fresh mountain air you've drawn deep into your lungs—Mother Nature, having already flaunted her beauty, decides to please you even more. Intricately colored butterflies flutter to and fro and from flower to flower, each exquisite bloom generously offering up its sweet fragrance. Bees buzz by, busily sampling the sweet nectar and carrying it off to distant places. As though to compliment the phenomenal array of activity going on around you, a medley of tunes begins to play: You hear the clicking and chatter of busy-bodied chipmunks and bushy-tailed ground squirrels as they scurry about foraging for food. Birds cheerfully chirp, their medley of happiness as evident as that of the other multitude of inhabitants of this hill who, though unseen, make their presence known.

In this moment, all call out to each other. What a choir!

You can't help but feel the powerful stirrings going on inside of you. You marvel at all this intoxicating splendor, and ponder what it must be like to be a butterfly, willfully following a sweet scent, or a bird free to surf the warm winds. You feel a kinship with all the other little creatures making their way through the day, most especially that little rodent playing hide-and-seek with the shadow overhead in hopes he doesn't become a hungry hawk's timely, tasty lunch.

Inner Peace—The Most Perfect Expression of Beauty

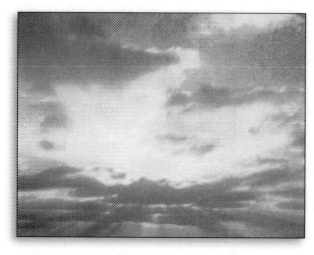

Make time to enjoy the awesome beauty of sunsets.

These are precious moments. In such moments we can't help but grasp that we live in a universe buzzing and humming with life—a life force in which all beings are dependent upon each other.

These moments are insightful. In these moments wherein the gentle whistling of the wind speaks louder than the laughter of friends or the experience of our victories and defeats, intuitively we are reminded to "drink in" the knowledge that our heart, mind, body and soul are at this moment "one"—and *perfect*.

And these moments are sacred. Lost in time, we are reunited with truths larger and more profound than events in our everyday lives. We live in a world of creation, one where a universal energy permeates all living matter. What a shame if we don't grasp the importance of being in harmony with that which is all around us.

Though your friends call out to you, as much as you love being in their presence, human words intrude on the power of this feeling of completeness. You realize this feeling is the best! It can hardly be improved upon. Having more friends, getting a new outfit, even having more dollars in your wallet— all seem unnecessary in this moment. A new hairstyle, or the latest shade of lipstick or nail polish cannot brighten your outlook more than the glow you feel when all is well on the inside.

Feeling complete, being at peace within, is the most *perfect* expression of beauty.

The Fountain of <u>True</u> Inner Beauty

I believe with all my heart that the feeling of being at peace and complete is an outcome of our faith. Faith is the eternal spring from which *true* inner beauty flows. One of the most beautiful women I've ever seen is Heather Whitestone, Miss America 1995—a shining example of the power of this spring. Devout in her faith and certain that her calling is to witness to the purpose of it, her deep inner harmony shines outwardly in a joy that leaps from her face to your heart. It is the innocent beauty of her soul, created by the anchor of her faith, that you see even before you notice Heather's striking physical beauty. Perhaps you have seen her on television commercials or speaking to youth around the country. Once you've seen this exquisite woman, you will *never, ever* forget her. Her outer beauty is undeniably breathtaking. But it is her inner radiance that is so incredibly captivating to the point that she is simply unforgettable.

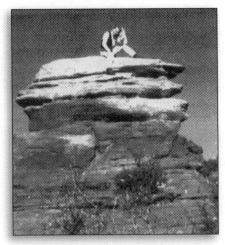

Make room in your life to spend quiet time—alone.

One on One— Alone or in a Crowd

Being together, talking, laughing and just sharing is a common experience that affirms we are a part of the greater whole of the human race. But just as we are a part of a vast human civilization, like a single star among the vast galaxy wherein each star has its own force to play out, we each journey through time alone, and we each experience it in our own way. We humans are each a single soul in search of meaning. We must feed our hearts. As much as we like and need our friends, no amount of exciting times with them can compensate or take the place of finding the meaning of our own existence. Even when with others, we experience our lives one on one. We will each

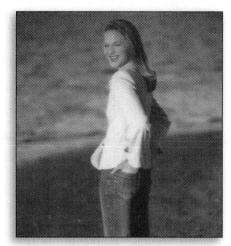

Embrace nature at the beach.

encounter times in our lives when we are faced with challenges we must cope with all alone.

Acknowledging a one-on-one relationship with a force greater than ourselves is the foundation of faith. Faith can provide us with leadership and strength, drawing upon sources that inspire and uplift us, as they tie us to the timeless truths of all humanity, truths that in our souls we know to be so.

The Source of Inner Strength and Guidance

An unending source of joy and peace, this ever available faith is also a source of strength and guidance—an anchor that sustains us not only when all is going well, but especially when we feel alone or overwhelmed. It offers comfort when no one else can—as many teens in the Columbine massacre discovered when for more than three hours they holed up in Columbine's choir office. Facing a terrorist wasn't the first time seventeen-year-old Cassie Bernall drew upon her faith. Once a troubled teen who did drugs, her faith became her reason for turning from the despair of drugs and helped her realign her life toward a purpose. Countless others have found this to be true as well. At the heart of most Twelve Step recovery programs, such as Al-Anon, Alcoholics Anonymous and others like them, spiritual principles stand as a point of hope to acquire the strength and direction to achieve and maintain freedom from destructive behavior. Experts have found that it is only by surrendering to the unconditional love of a Higher Power that most people "recovering" from serious addictions are able to live freely.

Soul Food: Your Faith

Because faith is so central to our wholeness, and it is this wholeness that gives us this inner harmony, a harmony that radiates from the inside out, we need to care for this vital source of genuine beauty. Your spiritual self needs nourishment.

Whatever your faith, feed your heart and soul by studying the doctrines of your religion and applying their meaning to your everyday life. Don't worry that you will be considered a prude. Just the opposite is true. Modeling faith is uplifting and inspirational to others. The example of Cassie Bernall's witnessing of her faith on that tragic last day of her life in Littleton, Colorado, galvanized teens nationwide to think about faith and its role in their lives. Rallies within nearly thirty states are now underway for teens to ponder their own respective faith and ways to serve it. Countless Internet sites are now devoted to teen faith, and fresh, new songs are penned heralding the role of faith in our lives.

Eavesdrop on the Universe: Experience the Mysterious

We may not always understand the workings of faith, but that doesn't make it any less real or valuable. Albert Einstein said, "The most beautiful thing we can experience is the mysterious." Sometimes faith is found on just such mysterious experiences. Check it out for yourself:

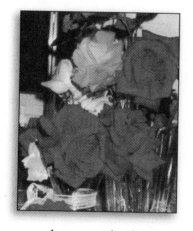

- Eavesdrop on the way the universe silently breathes its wonders into life. Plant three different kinds of flowers. Water them. Observe them as they grow. Notice how different and intricate each bloom is. Enjoy their beauty. Notice how a dry seed willfully grows into a thing of delicate beauty. Appreciate the mystery of life.

- Eavesdrop on the way the universe pulses with love. Watch the eyes of someone light up when they speak about someone they love. Observe the obvious joy and love of parents of a newborn when they talk about their baby. Watch the searing emotions apparent in the eyes of parents as they describe the joys and victories—or the trials, tribulations and defeats—of their teenager. Notice how deeply protective the bonds of love are. Marvel at the depth and power of such passion.

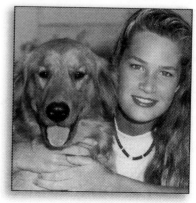

- Eavesdrop on the still, quiet way the universe unites you to all life. Contemplate the tug you've felt inside your heart to offer a smile to a stranger, to speak softly to a pet, to help someone in trouble, or to be kind, or simply to do the right thing. Why this *feeling* and what is its source? Then think of how good it made you feel when you responded to that inner calling. Recall the sense of purpose, of value and connection this contact and response ultimately brought you. Reflect on the mysterious unity that exists in being part of a much greater whole.

Believe that your life has a purpose, and that you have something to contribute. You are valued, wanted and needed. Allow your faith to nourish you in all times, good as well as difficult. Feel the power of it in your life. It is a potent source of a most radiant and luminous beauty.

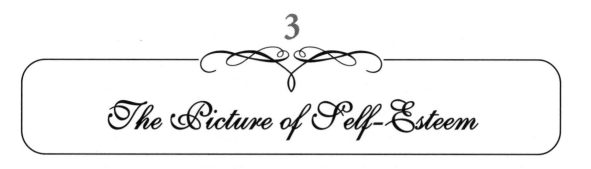

3

The Picture of Self-Esteem

Health comes from learning
to live in vibrant harmony with ourselves,
with the natural world, and
with one another.

—JOHN ROBBINS

The "Me" of Me

Have you noticed how some people are very comfortable being themselves? LeAnna Simons, one of my really good friends, is that way. People are always remarking, "LeAnna has such a nice 'presence' about her, such a positive 'sense of self.'" And they're right. LeAnna has good self-esteem.

Self-esteem is self-regard, how much you cherish and appreciate being you. It's the "price tag" you place on yourself. Are you a valuable commodity, or a "markdown"?

It's all about a *self* picture. Our price tag advertises for others what we think of ourselves—and they will pretty much treat us accordingly. Think of it: When you're shopping, don't you handle a $100 blouse a lot more carefully than a

$20 blouse? The way you communicate (your choice of words, your tone and style of relating, how well you listen), as well as how you present yourself (your appearance, your manners), are just a few of the many telltale signs of how much you value, honor and respect yourself. Psychologists say that self-esteem has a direct effect on all aspects of your health—mental, social and physical. Healthy self-esteem serves you well. Not so for low self-esteem. Teens with low self-esteem are more likely to do poorly in school, suffer from eating disorders and to engage in self-destructive behaviors, like smoking, drinking, doing drugs and being promiscuous.

Because the way you think of yourself is evident in everything you say and do, how you feel about yourself is often obvious to the people around you. What we think of ourselves becomes our "price tag."

"Just Me, Love Dan"

Because your self-regard is reflected in your behavior, other people can readily see what you think of yourself. In a workshop I conducted for teens some months ago, a seventeen-year-old guy told me that once when he wrote his girl-friend, Katerina, a letter and signed it "Just me, Love Dan" she gave the letter back to him, telling him she didn't like the way he signed it. "I'd like to think that I'm going out with someone who thinks more of himself than *just me,"* she informed him. "When you sign your letters, 'just me,' I take it to mean you don't think of yourself as very special, so *I* must not be all that special either."

You see, to Dan, Katerina was absolutely the best thing in the world. He treasured her and was honored and so happy to be going out with her. "Why on earth would you think that?" he asked, completely surprised at her words. "Because," Katerina replied, "if you don't think very much of you, how could you possibly be going out with a really great girl, like me? I'd like to think of myself that way—as a really special person. But if you don't think much of you, how can you be worthy of me? I mean, I don't want to go out with a guy who thinks of himself as 'nobody special.'"

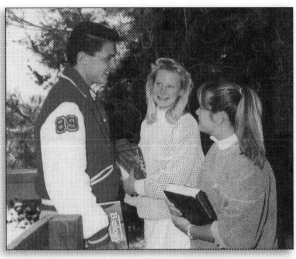

Good self-esteem makes for better friendships.

It's an interesting point. Obviously Dan's girlfriend thought Dan was special, *special* enough to be dating him, *special* enough to be her steady boyfriend. It made perfect sense to Katerina that her boyfriend should consider himself worthy enough for her. Because Katerina thinks of herself as a terrific girl, it's a put-down to Katerina for Dan to consider himself a "just me," a "nobody special."

"After thinking about it," Dan told me, "I realized Katerina was right. I decided to stop talking (and writing) about myself in a way that made me look as though I am not a person who appreciates how good it is to have Katerina for a girlfriend—and how good it is to have me as my own friend, someone I admire and speak well of. It was a valuable lesson. Just as I sign my letters to Katerina with 'Love, Dan' to let her know that my feelings for her are positive and loving, the words I say to me should be as positive and loving, too."

Self-Esteem: Building Beauty from the Inside Out

As Katerina explained to Dan, self-esteem shows how you feel about yourself. It's the level of your self-confidence—how bright, personable, caring, witty and wonderful you think you are. This self-picture affects how you care for your health and value your well-being; how meticulous you are in your grooming; the friends you choose; the goals you set and achieve. It also makes a major difference in how happy you are! [Happiness and a fun personality are always in style—see colorplates 18–21.]

There was a guy in my high school, Brent, who found it all too easy to belittle others. "Another bad hair day, Susan?" he'd snicker to a classmate of ours if her hair wasn't particularly as neat and well-groomed as she usually kept it. "Nothing zinc wouldn't cure," was a favorite phrase of his when a classmate had scored low on a test or quiz or done poorly on a homework assignment. This comment was usually followed by Brent waving his high marks or good score in the air for the other students to see. Brent always made others feel insignificant and pointed out how smart he was. Unfortunately Brent's proclamations of his good marks and talents always came at another's expense.

Every now and then someone would remark that Brent "really felt *sure* of himself." In fact, the opposite was true. If Brent had felt better about himself, then he wouldn't have found it necessary to be so critical of others.

With a healthy self-esteem, far from being conceited or self-centered, you have an authentic sense of self. This means you understand that you are human. You have good days. You have bad days. You have ordinary days. You are awesome and capable of greatness. You are vulnerable and will sometimes fail at things. Allowing both the ups and downs, taking the good with the bad, gives you a more realistic sense of self, a compassionate sense of self. If you can imagine and accept this range of traits within yourself, then you can imagine and accept this range within others. This is what it means to "understand" and "show consideration to" others.

The Benefits of a Healthy Self-Esteem

- The higher your self-esteem, the more accepting and honoring you are of yourself. You like yourself. You want you as a friend.

- The higher your self-esteem, the more you take care of yourself. Because you value your health and wellness, you do the things that protect them.

- The more you appreciate yourself, the less likely it is that you will compare yourself with others. Your measuring stick for judging yourself is *within*.

- The higher your self-esteem, the better able you will be to find ways to get along well with others. Teens with a healthy self-esteem form close relationships with people who respect and value them.

- The higher your self-esteem, the more likely you will treat others with respect and fairness, since self-respect is the basis of respect for others.

- The higher your self-esteem, the more you will attract others who enjoy their lives and are working to their potential. People with low self-esteem tend to seek low-self-esteem friends, who also think poorly of themselves.

- The higher your self-esteem, the better able you are to cope with the ups and downs of life. Teens with a healthy self-esteem have a realistic view of their strengths and weaknesses and maintain a positive attitude when they fail at a task.

- The higher your self-esteem, the more likely you will be to think about what you want out of life, the more ambitious you will be in going after it and the more likely you will be to achieve it.

- The higher your self-esteem, the more you will confront obstacles and fears, rather than avoid them. Low-esteem individuals see problems as grounds for quitting and often say to themselves, "I give up."

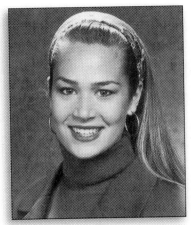

You can "see" a healthy self-esteem!

- The higher your self-esteem, the more able you are to recognize your own worth and achievements without a constant need for approval from others.
- The higher your self-esteem, the more responsibility you take for your own actions. When you recognize that you are off course, you are more likely to self-correct, to stop going in a negative direction and begin anew.
- The higher your self-esteem, the more willing you are to hang in there, even when the going gets tough. Because you persist, your chances for experiencing success are greater. The more success you experience, the less likely it is that you will feel devastated or deflated by periodic setbacks.
- The higher your self-esteem, the happier you are. And a happy person with a big smile is a beautiful person who makes other people want to be around her.

Can You Change Your Self-Esteem?

Yes. You can change your self-esteem, but it's not a yo-yo. You don't just wake up one day with a high self-esteem or a low self-esteem. It's not like having a good hair day and a bad hair day. On some days, it seems like your hair has a mind of its own and it won't do what you want no matter what, but self-esteem isn't like that.

Your self-esteem is the whole picture of how you see yourself. Experts say that this picture is the product of about a year's worth of "pictures." Here's the way it works. Let's say that you are an average student in math. For most of your ninth-grade year, you received Cs. If this is the case, when friends ask you if you are "good at math," chances are you will say, "average." So if you get an A on a test during this year when you see yourself as an average student, you will be very happy (or think it was "just luck"), but the one A is unlikely to change your mind about being an "average" student in math.

Now, let's say that you have been getting Cs for the first three months of ninth-grade math, and then, for the next three months you have been earning mostly As. How do you see yourself, as a C student or an A student? If you see yourself as earning As more and more consistently, your view of yourself as a C student is going to change. And that's the way it is with esteem. If the picture you had of yourself in the past was of someone who doesn't speak up for herself, as someone in the habit of putting herself down, of not having friends (you get the idea), but now you see yourself as working on your goals, as being a courteous and conscientious person who is slowly but surely gaining the respect of others (yourself included), then the image of yourself is changing.

What wonderful news! We can improve our self-esteem.

From Bad to Good, from Bad to Worse

Naturally there's a catch. Self-esteem can go from good to bad, too. Using the example above, things could be reversed. If you have been a good student in math for awhile, but for the last half-year things have changed and you are now getting lower and lower grades, then chances are you are going to lose confidence in yourself as being a good student in math class.

The same concept applies to your ideas of how attractive you are. Maybe your overall sense of your attractiveness up until now was pretty good. But then the stage of adolescence begins with all of its growth demands—enormous physical changes move your body from a child to an adult, accompanied by erratic mood shifts and ups and downs, highs and lows. All these new and puzzling changes can leave you wondering if you're okay and if you are all that attractive and desirable to others, especially if you're trying to get used to the "new you."

The news is still good: You can work to improve the image you have of yourself. This holds true in almost every area, whether it be your image of your body as healthy, fit and attractive, or your image of yourself as a student, a friend, or a son or daughter.

Because a healthy self-esteem is so important, caring for it is one of the most important things you can do. A healthy self-esteem is achieved by actively participating in your life in a meaningful way. For example, you make a pact with yourself to be your own best friend, and not to say or do those things that do not represent you. You take responsibility for your choices, actions and behavior. You work toward those goals that are important to you. You think about what you want out of life—and work toward bringing your ideals to life.

Self-esteem is a consequence of your actions. The more you set and achieve worthwhile goals in all areas of your life, the better you respect and honor yourself.

How to Improve Your Self-Esteem

Because self-esteem is so important, you need to know how to take care of yours. A healthy self-esteem is a result, a consequence of seeing yourself doing positive things in positive ways in five key areas:

1. Your sense of purpose
2. Your emotional security (intrinsic worth)
3. Your friendships and associations with others
4. Your safety
5. Your achievements (and sense of being a capable person)

Throughout this book, you'll learn more about how to care for yourself in each of these areas, but in a nutshell, here are the things you can do to have a "good reputation" with yourself.

- Believe that you have a right to live a happy and fulfilling life.

- Take good care of your body. Don't take risks that could put your safety and your health in jeopardy (such as using drugs and alcohol).

- Get to know and understand yourself and make friends with the face in the mirror. Treat yourself with respect. Don't put yourself down with sarcasm or hurtful words. (Others will take your lead and treat you as you treat yourself. Remember, *you* are the one setting this standard.)

- Make choices consistent with values you know to be good and right, those you can be proud to stand up for.

- Set worthy goals and strive to achieve them.

- Develop a "can-do" attitude, but accept that just as you have strengths, you have weaknesses. Everyone has both.

- Take time out regularly to be alone with yourself so that you can listen to yourself and ponder your inner thoughts and feelings. Cultivate activities you can enjoy by yourself, like crafts, reading or an individual sport. The goal is to become your very best friend, to truly enjoy your own company.

- Learn effective ways to manage the way(s) you respond to stress.

- Practice your faith. Faith is about the timeless truths and provides leadership to your heart and soul—the core of your being.

- Read broadly and expose yourself to great minds. This allows you to examine your own assumptions, and to grow and become wise. Refuse to narrow and close your mind so that assumptions are never examined.

• Reach out to others to talk about how things are going for you. You will find others know what you are talking about. They've been there. People around you understand and are willing to cut you some slack, especially if you are good-natured and courteous. It's only natural that sometimes you'll mess up. When this happens, admit it, talk about it, apologize for your shortcomings, and then vow to do better. This shows maturity. And you'll feel better about yourself and more confident in getting through the next "crisis"—and there will be many. That's just the way life is when you're a teen.

You Don't Have to Go It Alone

Learning how to cope effectively with your life can help you be a happy person—and that's the goal. But sometimes the stress and strains are simply too big for you to handle alone. Asking for help when you need it is a sign of strength and an attribute of inner beauty—and a mark of a person with good self-esteem.

Should you be facing struggles that seem overwhelming, rather than suffer alone or resort to doing things that are self-destructive, I urge you to confide in a best friend, as well as an adult you trust. (This is especially true in the case of physical or sexual abuse, suicidal feelings, eating disorders, depression, pregnancy or using drugs or alcohol.) Remember that parents, teachers and other professionals such as school nurses or counselors were once teens (and many are the parents of teens) and know what it feels like to be unsure of yourself, to have fears and anxieties about coping with life in general. It can be helpful to remember that if you have had a bad experience when an adult seemed aloof to your needs, or even broke your trust, this is generally the exception to the rule. Trust that adults have the best interest of teens at heart and want to help you make the best choices in dealing with the things going on in your life. **And here's a secret I'd like to let you in on.** It can be scary to tell your parents that you feel in over your head on something—like experimenting with drugs or drinking or suspecting you may be pregnant—for fear that they will be upset with you. The truth is, they probably will be upset in the beginning because they may be as overwhelmed and frightened as you. But even if you think they will be upset, even if you feel you have let your parents down, tell them anyway because once they work through their own fears and feelings, most always they will get to work to help you sort things out. After all, your well-being is their number-one concern, so brave their reaction and know that in the end, your parents usually are the ones who know what's best for you and will do all they can to help you. And once your parents are on board, they will help you see it through to the end. I know this. I've experienced it firsthand as a teen myself, and have had hundreds and hundreds of teens tell me how turning to their parents, as difficult as it may have been, was the best thing they could have done.

And remember, especially when life seems particularly stressful, it's time to be extra good to yourself—get adequate rest, eat properly and get the exercise your body needs to burn off tension. "Cool" is a decidedly wonderful aspect of beauty, one that begins on the inside and radiates out.

If You've Got It Together . . .

As you can see, a healthy self-esteem is pretty important to that "price tag" you set for yourself. When you have a healthy self-esteem, it is often so noticeable that it prompts others to remark, "You really have your act together!"

Why is self-esteem such a valued commodity? Because a positive sense of self is a sure contribution to your beauty. [See colorplate 9.]

4

From "Me" to "You"

*When we seek to discover the best in others, we
somehow bring out the best in ourselves.*

—WILLIAM ARTHUR WARD

Harmony: It Takes Two to Tango

Self-esteem is a focus on self and your own needs. Learning how to nurture yourself, being attentive to your own needs and interests, leads to a sense of being "in sync" within your life. This internal sense of confidence and peace provides a feeling of contentment and harmony. But excessive self-absorption creates a profound sense of loss, of alienation and isolation from ourselves. Like the expression goes, "No man is an island."

We need others.

As we grow in self-awareness and understand the importance of feeling at peace with ourselves, we move from concentrating solely on the self and its internal experience of harmony, to an outward sense of harmony with others. Having developed skills for seeing into yourself, and having learned to appreciate what you see, you can now apply these skills of "seeing into me," to "seeing into you." It's an important venture.

As we turn our focus outward, moving from "me" to "you" adds yet another dimension to our inner contentment. It makes us happy. The more *harmonious* the relationships we have with others, the greater our inner satisfaction—in a word, happiness.

What Makes You *Most* Happy?

What do you think is the greatest source of happiness for people? When you think about those times when *you* are truly happy and content, to what do you attribute it? Is it because you have just accomplished something, like acing a big test? Or is it because you are in a really "good space" with your family and friends?

In *Taste Berries for Teens,* a book I coauthored with my mother, we asked nearly six thousand teens "What makes you happy?" Teens of all ages and from diverse backgrounds said "feeling close to their friends and parents" was a source of their feeling content. As it turns out, the same thing is true for adults! In April of 1996, ABC television—in conjunction with an hour-long program on happiness—polled the American public, asking them, "What accounts for the greatest happiness in life?" Their answer? Close relationships. This was followed by control over one's life, challenging and fulfilling work, a sense of optimism, faith in God, and a sense of purpose. Money and material things—such as a great house or cars and such—did not show up in the top six on the list, contrary to what many might suspect.

For teens and adults as well, feeling close—a sense of community and connection—is a rich source of happiness.

The Bunny-Love Experiment

This connection with others is also good for our health! This was demonstrated accidentally in a research project using rabbits as subjects. Researchers couldn't understand why within a large pen of bunnies, noticeable differences surfaced in the bunnies after about a month or so of being together. Some bunnies appeared to be in better health than others; for example, their coats were thick and shiny. Some bunnies were more social and playful, while others began to withdraw, huddle alone or shy away from the others.

Because all bunnies were fed the same diet, scientists really couldn't account for the differences. Baffled, the directors of the research looked into it. What they discovered was an amazingly simple explanation. Each and every day, a night lab worker had been playing with some of the bunnies, giving certain ones his attention and affection as he was cleaning the lab.

Once the researchers learned this, they separated the bunnies into two groups, this time deliberately giving certain rabbits more attention and affection than the others. Sure enough, the bunnies receiving the affection and attention once again showed better overall health, and were more social—romping more playfully with each other than the others. Obviously, TLC (tender loving care) is good for a bunny's health and sense of play!

Like bunnies, people "thrive" on attention and care, too.

Getting—and Giving—All the TLC You Need

Think about those people who are your anchors, those you can count on to be there for you, whether to cheer you on or to help you mend an aching heart. For me it's my parents, friends and grandparents—especially my Grandma Burres. I think of her often, and when I do, usually she'll call. When I call her, she'll almost always say to me, "Oh, 'Jennicans'" (one of her three nicknames for me—and one that only she is allowed to use!), "I was just thinking of you!" Connecting with my grandma is always a good feeling. But she also has a way about her of being so solid, so strong, so able to make me feel whole.

When I was growing up, at those times when my mother was "out of juice," as she would say, she'd go to spend a day or two with her parents. "Spending even a day with them is like going to the well!" she would report. "Whenever I'm in need of mothering, no one puts me back together quite as my mom and dad do!" As a child, I didn't really understand what she meant when she said

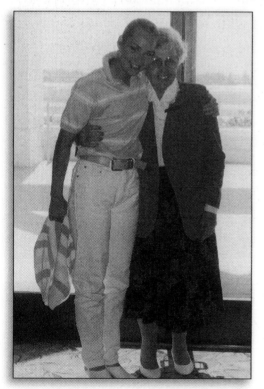

Unconditional love: my grandmother and me

this, but I do know that when my mother returned home, she was peaceful, joyful and serene. Being with her parents provided her with a source of strength unlike the other people she needed in her life. Now I fully understand the importance of being with people who make us feel good about ourselves, who provide us with a safe place to share our innermost thoughts and needs, and who love us unconditionally. My grandmother is that special to me, as is my mother. There are others of course, but I realize the *importance* of these two significant people in my life.

Family—Cookies and Milk for the Heart

Family is a most important source of TLC. As a teenager, you may not always feel that your parents are a number-one source, but *usually* they are. I know when I'm at odds about something with my mom or dad, even though I act strong and pretend it's not that big of a deal, the truth is, it's very upsetting to me. When I was in high school (and still, even now at twenty-five), an argument with my parents was dis-heartening. If I disagree with them, and even if I'm sure I'm right in going with a choice I've made over another one they've counseled me to select, I feel uneasy, like there's a piece of my life that isn't in harmony. And of course, that disharmony is upsetting. My parents and I have a close relationship, and I love and respect them, so when we're on the outs, when there's discord, it doesn't feel good.

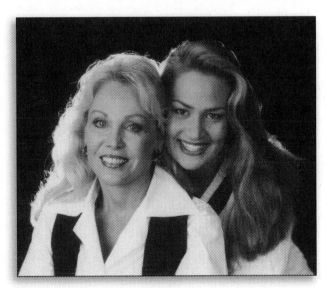

Heartstrings: my mother and me

My friends feel the same. Jaime, a seventeen-year-old friend said it this way: "If I'm in an argument with my parents, it isn't like I can go to school and just forget about it. I'll be sitting in class, not really paying attention to what is going on because I'll be off in my mind, still thinking about the argument. Rather than concentrating on what the teacher is saying, I'm still involved: *What* were my parents thinking? *Why* did they say what they did (or didn't)?

Then I wonder why *I* said what I did—or why I didn't say what I should have! And then I try to decide on a good time and a good way to reopen a conversation with them so I can go where I wanted, or get what I wanted or have what I wanted in the first place!

"So I sit in class, planning a new strategy, and playing through every possible response—several times. Of course, this means that I'm still not paying attention to what's going on in class. This upsets me too, so then I get worked up all over again. Sometimes I take out my frustration on my teachers, or my friends by being impatient with them, or I pass my anxiety off on them—even though I don't mean to. I'm not the only one this happens to. My friends feel upset too when it happens to them. What I'm learning is that feeling close to my parents is important to me. I want to have a good relationship with them."

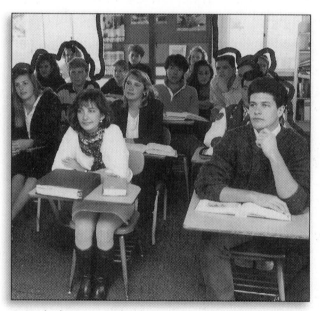
Strive for harmony with others.

Many teens feel like Jamie. And many teens also want to be close to their siblings. Believe it or not, brothers and sisters are our number-one fans. My friend Alicia and her younger sister bicker between themselves all the time, but when it comes to defending each other, no one is more loyal than they are to each other. So, take good care of your relationship with your family and work to be in a harmonious relationship with them. Of all my friends, those who have good relationships with their families are happier than those who are constantly on the outs with them. As for me, I always feel happiest when I'm in a "good place" with my family—and with my friends.

Friends—Pizza for Life!

What would life be like if you didn't have good friends? For me, I can't even imagine it! Like teens everywhere, I rely on harmony with my friends as an important source of contentment.

For me, a good friend is someone I can count on, someone with whom I can relax and just hang out, have fun and share my innermost thoughts—deep, dark secrets, lofty and noble goals, or my hopes, joys and fears. I know a friend is a good friend when I feel that with her it is okay—a safe space—to share my deepest thoughts and needs—without worry of being judged, criticized or made to feel silly for feeling the way I do. Friends cheer each other on, laugh and cry together, and just plain commiserate and listen to each other. That's why friends are friends.

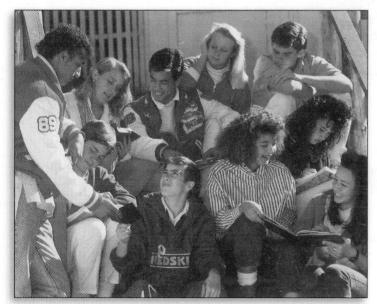

Having friends is a source of inner happiness.

Friends help you to grow into being who you are and allow you to reveal those parts of yourself that you may be meeting for the first time. What a wonderful gift. From coping with the death of a loved one to dealing with the everyday ups and downs of life—like sharing a secret too good to keep, or mourning a breakup with a special someone—friends are important in our lives.

Having people who are "there for us" as a source of strength, support and rejuvenation is not only special, but important. Take a moment to think about who provides this source of comfort to you. Hold these relationships close to your heart and protect them by staying in touch and showing your support, remembering to offer them comfort in return.

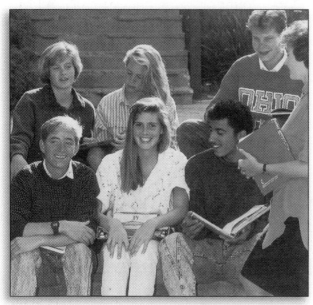

Help others feel good about themselves.

TLC Is a Two-Way Street

The key to being a good friend is fairly simple: It's reaching out to show others you are thoughtful and considerate, and a person who strives to create harmony among others. How? By seeing the good in others and letting them know how much they mean to you.

When you help others feel good about themselves, you help them see you as someone special to them. If you want to test this principle, recall a time when someone made a comment that made you feel good about yourself. For example, just recently I had some red highlights added to my hair. A girl I work with noticed and said, "Oh, Jennifer! Your hair color is positively fabulous; it looks just great on you!" Her comment made me feel "positively fabulous" all day.

Share the joy.

There are many ways you can share good feelings with others. For example, if you notice a friend or classmate has a new haircut or is wearing her hair differently and it looks really good, you can say, "I really like your new hairstyle.

It looks great on you!" If a friend (or parent or teacher) is in an especially good mood or is feeling excited about something, you can say, "Being in a good mood sure looks great on you!" If a friend or classmate has been working out, cheer them on with a good word of encouragement: "That jogging you've taken up is really paying off! You look really good." If someone has just taken a leap to wearing a new style of clothes or color of makeup that works well for them, tell them about it. If someone is having a bad day, stop and listen. Show empathy.

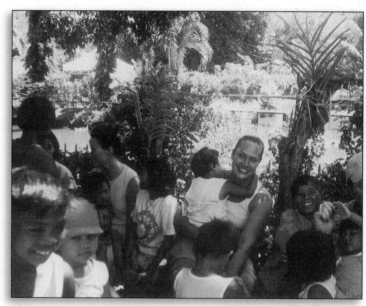

Helping others feel good about themselves will not only win you friends, but it will make you feel better about yourself. Try it and see! Open doors for people young and old, offer to help, say a kind word, pick up a piece of trash

With new friends on an Airline Ambassadors/United Nations mission to deliver humanitarian aid to an orphanage in the Philippines.

even though it wasn't you who discarded it. Volunteer in your community. Be a person who likes people. We live in a world with others. I love a saying from one of my mother's books, *Taste-Berry Tales:* "It is our obligation—as much as it is our honor—to help others see their lives in a positive light." I believe that. I know from experience that helping others is a most important way to see yourself as a loving and generous person. And feeling good about yourself is a positive contribution to your beauty.

"Play with Him"

From saving a lizard to building homes for Habitat for Humanity, there are many ways to get involved in the lives of others. Some of these can be as simple as being good to the people we meet in our everyday lives. I remember being with my mother on a television interview for a recent book. Actress Annie Potts was also a guest on the show. When asked how she managed professional life along with being the mother of three young children, she listed several things that helped her, one of them being her children's looking out for each other. One of her remarks especially stood out. She said, "I tell my children to love each other, and then I take my older son aside and say, 'Be good to your little brother. *Play* with him.'" When I heard that, I thought, how loving—and how simple. Playing with his little brother when their mother was away was the ultimate show of taking a loving, caretaking role in the responsibility of seeing that the little boy was a happy little camper when Mommy was gone.

Believe that others need you. If ever you doubt it:

- Help someone who is ill, infirm or broken-hearted. Feel their vulnerability and hold it close to your heart. Feel how good it is to provide strength when another needs it.

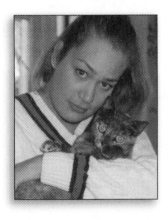

- Assist someone. If you see someone drop something, offer help gathering things. Watch the gratitude on that person's face.

- Call out in a friendly, comforting tone to a stray, lost or wounded animal. Feel the tug of your heart, and the tear within your eyes, as you offer compassion and extend human caring for the creatures nature has provided for our overseeing and protecting. Diligently care for your own pet. Allow yourself to feel the love your pet gives to you.

- Compliment others, even those you don't know, on how nice they look, whether it be the smile on their face, or the clothes they are wearing.

In doing these things, you'll find goodwill produces harmony. Inner harmony is a most luminous facet of beauty. There's nothing more radiant than an inner harmony that displays itself in sparkling eyes, a friendly smile and a sense of self that is generous enough to care about others.

5

The Beauty of Purpose and Passion

Doing quality work—that's what brings you self-respect.

—Sadie Delany, age 107, first African American woman
to teach home economics in New York City schools

Patricia Hill Burnett

In the photo of me with my friend Patricia Hill Burnett (author of *True Colors: An Artist's Journey from Beauty Queen to Feminist,* [see page 51 and colorplate 39]) notice how vibrant she looks: Her smile is generous, her eyes sparkle, she is sitting tall and looking directly at you! Dressed impeccably as always, in stylish and vibrantly colored clothes, and wearing beautiful jewelry that compliments her apparel, she is a picture of beauty. All of this gives off an air that here is a smart and classy woman, a woman who is in command of herself. And she is!

A large part of Patricia's vibrancy comes from her active involvement in her life—and work. And this is one of the great secrets of real beauty. A prime source of "confidence" and "motivation" and "sass" and "spunk" and "vitality"— all traits we admire and revere in others—emanates from *feeling purposeful.*

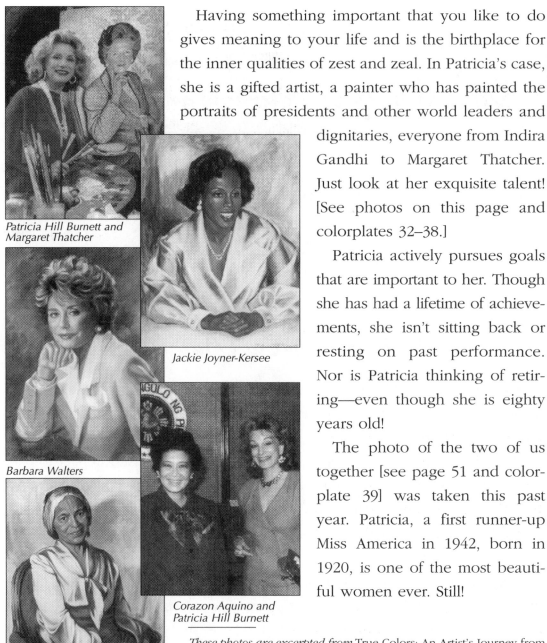

Patricia Hill Burnett and Margaret Thatcher

Jackie Joyner-Kersee

Barbara Walters

Corazon Aquino and Patricia Hill Burnett

Rosa Parks

Having something important that you like to do gives meaning to your life and is the birthplace for the inner qualities of zest and zeal. In Patricia's case, she is a gifted artist, a painter who has painted the portraits of presidents and other world leaders and dignitaries, everyone from Indira Gandhi to Margaret Thatcher. Just look at her exquisite talent! [See photos on this page and colorplates 32–38.]

Patricia actively pursues goals that are important to her. Though she has had a lifetime of achievements, she isn't sitting back or resting on past performance. Nor is Patricia thinking of retiring—even though she is eighty years old!

The photo of the two of us together [see page 51 and colorplate 39] was taken this past year. Patricia, a first runner-up Miss America in 1942, born in 1920, is one of the most beautiful women ever. Still!

These photos are excerpted from True Colors: An Artist's Journey from Beauty Queen to Feminist, *by Patricia Hill Burnett. Momentum Books Ltd., 1995. ©Patricia Hill Burnett. Reprinted with the permission of Patricia Hill Burnett. [See colorplates 32–38.]*

People like Patricia show us the importance of purposeful activity in our lives. It's part of what gives her such a sense of presence. I have always believed that a goal of work is to be able to make our joys our job, and Patricia has done just that. Patricia is an example of radiance that stems from her

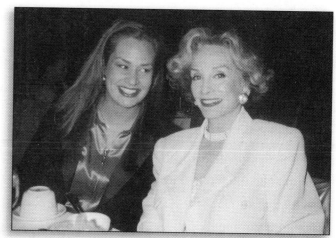

Patricia Hill Burnett and me

work as a source of satisfaction. When you are busy working toward something important, you feel purposeful.

Setting and achieving worthwhile goals is the key.

A Goal Is Like a Road Map

A goal is like having a map. If you know the direction you should be heading, you know where to focus your time and energy. Channeling your efforts in a single direction can keep you on track so that you actually get to your destination. How many times have you heard the expression, "I got sidetracked"? Goals keep you on track so you can accomplish your dreams. You know where you should be spending your time, and you have made plans to do the things you need to do to accomplish your desires. For example, suppose that you are going to run in a mile-long race. If you don't record on your calendar the date of the race, and then make a plan to assure that you do well in it—like eating the right foods, getting into shape, and warming up before the race—you just might tumble out of bed one morning and say, "Gee, I can't believe the race is today!" If you'd not made plans to do well in it, you may just feel awful when you are through—assuming you do finish!

Here are some helpful tips for setting goals:

1. Be specific in your goals. Goals that are specific, as opposed to ambiguous, provide better direction. For example, rather than, "Start working out," say, *"I'm going to exercise three times a week."*

2. Set a timeline and target dates for accomplishment. For example, *"I'm going to exercise each Monday and Thursday in my physical education class and go to the workout center with my mom on Saturdays."*

3. Break your goal into manageable parts. We call these subgoals. For example:

    Goal: To get adequate sleep each night.

    Subgoal: Will not drink caffeinated soft drinks at night.

    Subgoal: Will not play rock or heavy metal CDs at least one hour before going to bed.

    Subgoal: Get started on my homework right after school instead of waiting until the last minute.

4. Break your goals into realistic and manageable timelines so that you know what you should be doing and when. For example:

    Major Goal: To buff up.

    Subgoal: To tone my muscles.

    Monthly Goal: Work out ten times.

    Weekly Goals: Commit to a rigorous workout in gym class each Monday and Wednesday.

    Work out at the Family Fitness Center on Saturday with Mom (or a friend).

Take my dog Bowser for a ten minute run (or walk) after school instead of goading my little sister to do it for me.

5. Put your goals in writing. Doing so helps you clearly identify what you want, and it increases your personal commitment to your goals.

6. Keep a copy of your goal plan in sight and refer to it often. For example, if your goal is to exercise each Monday, Thursday and Saturday, tape a copy of that goal on the inside of your notebook, so you won't schedule yourself to do something else instead—like make plans with friends that keep you from your goal! If your goal is to stop eating junk food, put that goal on the refrigerator and maybe on the inside of your notebook so that when you pass the snack dispenser you will be more easily swayed to purchase an apple instead of a candy bar.

Guidelines for Setting Goals

It's really not enough to have one goal, nor is it realistic to have twenty goals and to think that you will actually accomplish all of them. Six categories of goals are shown below, with an added "other" area so you can create any other category you might want to work on. If you have one goal and one sub-goal in each area, you will have more than enough to do; yet you will not be so overwhelmed that you simply abandon doing the things you would like to achieve. Write down your goal and the primary subgoal in each category.

Creating Goals of Your Own

Relationships

(Goals in your relationships with parents, friends, teachers, others.)

Goal: _____

Subgoal: _____

Learning and Education

(What would you like to know more about? What skills do you want to

develop? To what formal education do you aspire?)

Goal: _____

Subgoal: _____

Job or Career Satisfaction

(Goals for getting a job or for preparing for what you want to do as a career.)

Goal: _____

Subgoal: _____

Leisure-Time Pursuits

(Goals for your leisure time and activities: hobbies, sports and other interests
you want to develop.)

Goal: _____

Subgoal: _____

Status and Respect

(To which groups do you want to belong? To what extent do you want to be respected by others? From whom do you want respect?)

Goal: _____

Subgoal: _____

Spiritual Growth

(Goals for peace of mind, your search for spiritual meaning.)

Goal: _____

Subgoal: _____

Others

(A goal that may not fit into the other categories, but is important to you.)

Goal: _____

Subgoal: _____

The More I Try, the Luckier I Get: Achievement Is a Source of Satisfaction

The more you accomplish your goals, the greater your sense of satisfaction. [See colorplates 22–23 and 25–26.] The greater your sense of satisfaction, the greater your sense of self. The greater your sense of self, the happier you are. The happier you are, the greater your inner beauty. And as you've learned throughout this book, that inner beauty keeps bubbling until it comes to the surface!

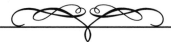

UNIT TWO
Health, Fitness and Nutrition

Good for the body is the work of the body,
and good for the soul is the work of the soul, and
good for either is the work of the other.

—HENRY DAVID THOREAU

Inventory: The Body You've Always Dreamed Of!

Do you like your body? What if you could have a little more of this, a little less of that? From your nose to toes, what changes would you make?

Head and Face: **Change I would make:**

❏ Hair color   _____

❏ Eye color   _____

❏ Forehead   _____

❏ Nose   _____

❏ Lips   _____

❏ Teeth   _____

❏ Chin   _____

❏ Ears   _____

❏ Neck   _____

Upper Body: Change I would make:

❏ Shoulders   _____

❏ Breasts   _____

❏ Arms   _____

❏ Hands   _____

❏ Fingers   _____

❏ Length of torso   _____

❏ Waistline   _____

Lower Body: Change I would make:

❏ Stomach   _____

❏ Hips   _____

❏ Buttocks   _____

❏ Thighs   _____

❏ Legs   _____

❏ Knees   _____

❏ Calves   _____

❏ Ankles   _____

❏ Toes

Overall: **Change I would make:**

❑ Height   _____

❑ Weight   _____

❑ Figure   _____

❑ Body build   _____

Did you wish you could make many changes, or only one or two? Or, do you like your body just as it is? If you said you would make changes, which ones seem most important to you? For example, if you said you wouldn't mind being a little taller, and prefer feet in the "perfect size," which is a stronger preference: to be taller or "perfect size" feet?

Probably we all would like to have a little more of this and a little less of that; it's natural to have a wish list. It helps to understand *why* we want to. To help you get a better look at this, go back over your list, and see if you can nail down a reason for your wanting "a little more of this, a little less of that." Is it based on the way your friends look, or something else entirely? Understanding yourself is an important part of accepting and loving yourself for who and what you are.

In this unit, you'll see how and why we girls think of our bodies as we do, as well as learn how to best care for your body from the inside out, so that it meets the most important test of all: *your* sense of its beauty. Because, when it comes right down to it, it's important that we make friends with ourselves, that we accept and love who we are, even without making changes.

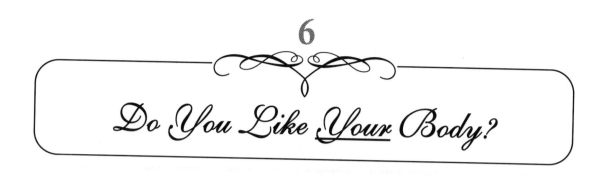

6

Do You Like Your Body?

*If anything is sacred, the
human body is sacred.*

—WALT WHITMAN

A recent poll surveyed a thousand adolescent girls asking them if they "liked their bodies." Only 14 percent of the girls polled answered "Yes." All the others said "No." If the poll is a representative of all teenage girls, that means that 86 percent of young women don't like their bodies. How unfortunate.

Sadly, I think the survey may have merit. Most of my friends in junior high and high school wished they were either taller or shorter, and wanted to either lose weight, or gain weight. Some with smaller breasts wished their chests were bigger, while those who had developed larger breasts said they wished they were less endowed. Some with curly hair wanted straight hair, while those with straight hair said they'd gladly trade their straight locks for a little natural curl. My issue was my feet. My feet were so big, I told my friends that I'd go out with a guy only if his shoe size was bigger than mine!

It seemed to me that just about all of us girls had a "wish list" of things we would like to change in one way or another when it came to our bodies. And you know, we were quite sure that practically all the guys we knew wanted to be taller and to have bigger muscles, but not one of them ever admitted it. Never ever did we hear a boy openly complain or express discontent about his body.

Why don't we girls appreciate our bodies more than we do? Could it be that we:

- Compare ourselves to the media image of the supermodel—an extraordinarily tall, rail-thin waif with perfect features and a flawless complexion, glamorous hair impeccably styled in the latest trend, and dressed in the newest fashion—a near-impossible standard to achieve in real life, so we feel inadequate, inferior in comparison?

- Allow the insensitive and critical comments made by a few of our peers to influence the way we see ourselves?

- Don't know how to accentuate or play up our best features while downplaying or offsetting those we don't like as much, especially those that cannot be changed—such as our height or bone structure?

- Don't take care of ourselves—like adhering to a healthy diet and exercising regularly—and so we are not as healthy as we could be?

We girls need to understand the pressures that influence how we see ourselves and make the choice to care for ourselves in healthy ways.

Pressures Influencing How Much You Like Your Body

I've Got to Be (Barbie Doll) Perfect

I remember a game my friends and I played in junior high when we girls were at a slumber party. It was called "Pick a Part," and we each picked a good "part" belonging to another girl. I wanted Tami's nose; she wanted my legs. Karen wanted Suzee's chest, while Suzee wanted Karen's chest. I always found this "game" insightful: While some of the "owners" didn't especially appreciate or like a certain part, others would have gladly traded with that person *because* we found the body part they didn't like *desirable*—and wouldn't mind having it for ourselves.

What is your standard of "perfect"? If you could describe the "perfect you" what would that be? I have friends who—because they compare themselves to looking like the "perfect model," as in the retouched photo of a magazine image (often a computerized image)—judge themselves harshly. The model in the magazine is an unrealistic standard. Don't buy into the "one size fits all" ideal when it comes to sizing up your beauty.

While the media may sometimes seem to be saying otherwise—"perfect" is pretty subjective. What is appealing to some people may not be to others. My friend Lena, who is Mexican American, loves to watch the music videos on Latin American television stations. "Latin Americans are so-o-o beautiful!" she exclaimed to me after watching one particular awards show. "In Latin American communities, round hips and having a little meat on your bones is considered sexy, very appealing—much more acceptable than where I go to school. I'm sure I'm considered ten to fifteen pounds overweight by my classmates, but in my family and in my community, I'm the perfect size." Lena's comment has merit. Beauty is impossible to stereotype. What one culture finds "most beautiful" is sure to be different from what another finds most appealing.

For the most part, "perfect" is determined by our own reference point. If six-feet, three-inch champion volleyball player Gabrielle Reece's daughter were to start kindergarten and find her female teacher was five foot five, would she see her mother as tall, or her teacher as short? And which would she most likely assume to be the more desirable height? Probably she would consider her mother's height more "beautiful."

If beauty is in the eyes of the beholder, let yourself be that beholder when it comes to your own standard of beauty. It's a real key to feeling good about who you are.

Caring for yourself means not falling victim to comparing your body to someone else's. Believe me, I know how this is easy to say and difficult to practice, especially when teens are constantly bombarded with the message that we *must* be "beautiful," and then blitzed with the products that will make us "beautiful." The message seems to imply that if we are the right height and size, and if we acquire the right things—the *right* makeup, the *right* clothes, the *right* accessories and so on—we, too, will look like Barbie. And this media-hyped, image-saturated message comes with the warning that should we fail to do this, we will never get a date, never have friends, never get the job of our dreams. Never . . . never . . . never. It's endless.

All these messages can be harmful to our sense of self and to appreciating our own individual brand of beauty. It's not as if we come off an assembly line, all resembling each other. We're all sizes, shapes and colors. You've seen it for yourself: One eighth-grade girl may be five feet, seven inches tall, and another four feet, seven inches. One girl may have brown eyes; another has green eyes. One may have a large bone structure, the other small and delicate bones. One may have an oval face, another a heart-shaped face. How silly to think there is a "perfect," a standard other than our own.

There are many forms of beauty. The goal is to appreciate yours.

Others Will Like Me Better If . . .

Friends and classmates can be tough critics. There will be those who feel they have the right to criticize or make snippy comments about how you dress, the way you look, your hairstyle, or the size or shape of your body. Don't allow their remarks—no matter how inconsiderate, rude or hurtful—to cause you to stop being your own best friend. I'm not saying that wanting others to think you're cool isn't important, because it is. But it's also important not to do those things that put your health and well-being at risk just to fit someone else's standard of cool.

You sometimes think, "I'll have more friends, or win so-and-so's friendship or be liked more if only I . . ." Fitting the mold of someone else's ideal is self-defeating. It's erroneous to believe that you will be better liked, more popular, or win the approval of the most popular boy or girl if only you would lose weight, or gain weight, or were taller or shorter, or had a great tan—or whatever. There will always be those who think you would look better if you were more of this or less of that. Trying to please yourself is hard enough without adding the burden of pleasing others.

There's something else you need to consider, too. Our peers may say things just to say things, or to "get to us," and sometimes, just as a way of relating—even flirting. Boys often don't know how to pay a compliment. They get embarrassed and when they mean to say, "You have a pretty smile," they may in fact blurt out, "What's with the big grin?" I had a boy say this to me once, and I remember thinking he thought I had a big mouth. He made similar off-the-wall statements for a full semester. I shied away from him as much as I could. When finally a girlfriend of mine told me she had heard through the grapevine—from the guy's sister (who was one of my friend's best friends)—that this boy was "madly in love" with me, you can only imagine how very surprised I was. Besides not taking everything you hear too seriously, when you start to worry too much about what others think, remind yourself that other than a few good friends, from the moment you get out of high school you will rarely see those people again. On the other hand, the way you've treated your health will stay with you year after year.

Play Today, Pay Tomorrow: Health Is Forever

The most important friend and protector your body can have—and the one who is with your body right up to the end—is you. Don't abuse it by doing things that will put your health in jeopardy. Take good care of yourself.

I'll never forget a comment made by my teacher one day in my health education course. "For better or for worse," she instructed, "the way you take care of yourself catches up to you." It wasn't until shortly after I was out of high school that I understood the meaning of her comment. The more I was around my friends, the more I could see the effects—the wear and tear—of their lifestyles in relationship to how they took care of themselves. For example, "Sam"—short for Samantha—is a friend of mine who works as a counter agent for a major airline. She works a four o'clock to eleven o'clock night shift at the airport, a job she's held for five years. It used to be that when she got off work, she would look up her friends and party until early morning. Then she would catch a couple of hours of sleep and be off to work again by four o'clock. Sam was twenty when I first met her. No one I knew was as party-hearty as Sam! And it shows. Already she has fine lines around her eyes from years of squinting because she smokes, and her skin looks sallow from it as well. And she has dark circles around her eyes from lack of sleep. She hasn't worked out since her days in high school, and she is out of shape and has gained weight because of it. She looks so much older than her twenty-five years.

The good news is that Sam is changing her ways. "I'm finding that staying out late and partying as often as I do is making it more difficult to function at work," she recently told a group of us girls having lunch. "And I'm beginning to gain weight because I don't eat properly, nor do I get enough exercise. And I really feel it. I just don't have the energy I did even a year ago."

I can understand that. Traveling from time zone to time zone as I sometimes do in my work seems more wearing to me now that I am twenty-five than it did when I was twenty-one! Although I refuse to admit that it's because I'm getting older, I do know that the way I take care of myself catches up with me. It used to be that I could get up early, work all day, stay up late, and be up early again—all seemingly without hurting my ability to be alert, energetic and conquer my day. Now, I need more sleep if I'm to meet the demands of my schedule. I also need to eat a balanced diet regularly, and I need to get to the gym to work out if I am to keep my body functioning at a high level. I still do my share of late nights and partying, and my work is demanding. But at least I'm more aware of the price my body pays for the strains I inflict on it. So I make an effort to take care of myself.

Even if it's natural to take your youth and good health for granted—don't. Take good care of you.

"Buffing Up" Begins on the Inside

When you were younger your parents saw to it that you ate well and got enough sleep. Their job as parents was to see to it that you had regular dental and medical checkups and that your growth and development were progressing in accordance with those of other kids your age. While your parents still oversee these things, there's no better time than adolescence to tune in to your body and to concern yourself with your own well-being.

Being healthy and fit begins with an attitude that says, "I want to be healthy and fit—so I'm going to take good care of myself." Taking responsibility for your well-being is a very different attitude from "I want to look great." There's an important distinction between the two. I have a good friend, for example, who took the ribbing of her friends in stride when they took up smoking, and she refused to smoke—even though they relentlessly tried to get her to join in. And I know for a fact that two of the girls who are a part of that clique didn't want to become smokers but allowed themselves to be bullied into smoking, and now both have developed the habit. One girl is up to two packs a day! I know another girl who would do almost anything to be thin. This included taking diet pills, because her friends were, even though these put her health at risk. Don't ever do those things that are abusive to your body. Feeling great and looking good is important, but never at the expense of your health.

Be good to yourself. Treat your body like it's your best friend *for life*.

From Nose to Toes: The Amazing Body Machine

"My body is constantly changing," sixteen-year-old Sandi Simon told me in a recent workshop I conducted for teens. "I want to know when the body I see in the mirror is going to be the body I'll have for good. *When* will my body be *done* changing?" As Sandi has discovered, in addition to keeping up with the external demands of their owners, our bodies are also busy with their own agenda.

With precision timing, our bodies carry out a series of tasks (all predetermined according to a biological time frame) designed to move the body from one stage of development to another. Be it the time to cut your first tooth or time to cut wisdom teeth, be it time for you to start your menstrual cycle or to start menopause, your body is in a continual process of doing those things that move you from a child to a senior. These life cycles are the automatic work of the body. Such is the nature of life.

Your body is an *amazing* machine. Respect all that it does to run efficiently.

Honoring "The Temple"

Several girlfriends and I were about to order a quick lunch from a fast-food drive-thru. "Bria, do you want an order of French fries with your chicken salad?" Chelsea asked. Bria was the only one who hadn't ordered fries. "No," she replied. "I never put fries in the temple." "The what?" Chelsea asked. "The temple—my bod," Bria replied. Bria has a good point. Given that French fries—as delicious as they are—probably aren't the world's best health food for your body, she was wise to opt for not eating them.

Your body is a living organism. As such, it needs adequate food, exercise and rest to go about its business of functioning properly. Sometimes it's not until we get sick (such as having a cold or the flu) or get hurt (such as spraining a muscle or pulling a ligament) that we realize how much we take our body's functioning for granted. Remember how much it hurt when you pulled a muscle playing a quick game of tag with your friends? Keep your body in the best condition you can.

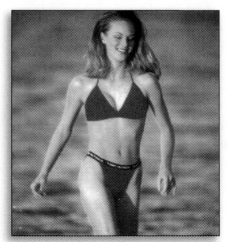
Keep your body in the best condition you can.

Taking care of yourself is about honoring your body and respecting all the demands placed on it. Just think of all that we ask of it. There's the pressure of keeping up with the tasks of daily life: work and play, school, part-time jobs, sports, hanging out with our friends, family life. Regardless of your hectic schedule or the amount of stress and strain you place upon your body, you expect it to go where you want when you want, and to perform with the necessary energy level you desire. These are big expectations. Don't make the body's job tougher than it already is.

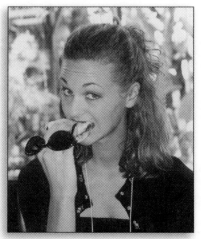

Believe me, I know how important it is to look great and feel well when you are with your friends, especially in the teen years when you spend almost your entire time with classmates and friends. It is important to fit in and to feel like one of the group. It's a wonderful feeling to be liked and accepted because you are seen as a part of the "in" crowd. But you must never compromise your health in the process. Always do those things that support your good health and wellness.

Go for good health!

Never sell out on you. Remember, your body is *yours,* and it's beautiful. Good health must never be taken for granted.

Making your health and well-being a priority means eating a balanced diet, getting enough rest and adequate exercise, and having a support system of family and friends to comfort and reassure you when you feel unsure or insecure about the many changes adolescence is sure to bring. These next chapters will show you how to better achieve all these things.

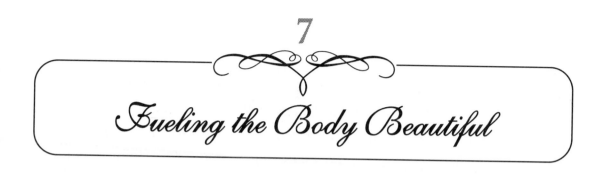

7

Fueling the Body Beautiful

*It's better to look ahead and prepare
than to look back and regret.*

—JACKIE JOYNER-KERSEE,
OLYMPIC TRACK-AND-FIELD CHAMPION

Food Is the Body's Fuel

Pop quiz: Name the last five foods you ate. Uh-oh! Were they Fritos, Coke, candy bar, Big Mac and fries? Your diet and nutrition play a key role in your overall health and wellness from how you look and feel to how well you can resist disease, even how well you perform mentally and physically. Good health depends on a balanced diet, on getting all the nutrients, vitamins and minerals your body needs to function properly. Any diet that emphasizes one type of food (protein, fat, carbohydrates, vegetables) to the exclusion of other foods may be very harmful to the body.

A deficiency of certain vitamins, minerals and nutrients can upset body chemistry, leaving you tired and prone to illness. A constant diet of Cokes, French fries and hamburgers, for example, will not sustain your body. Even the fast-food places understand this and feature milk and salads on the menu.

When your body lacks essential nutrients, it cannot function properly.

In all, your body needs about forty-seven different nutritional substances to sustain itself. Vegetables, whole-grain or enriched cereals and breads, a form of protein (such as beans or lean meat), and milk help the body function properly. The essential food groups considered vital for robust health include the meat group: meat, poultry, fish, dry beans, eggs, nuts and peanut butter; the dairy group: milk, yogurt, cheese, cottage cheese and ice cream. The vegetables and fruits group; and breads, cereals and pastas.

Food Guide Pyramid

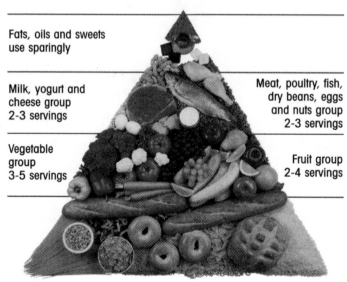

Fats, oils and sweets
use sparingly

Milk, yogurt and
cheese group
2-3 servings

Meat, poultry, fish,
dry beans, eggs
and nuts group
2-3 servings

Vegetable
group
3-5 servings

Fruit group
2-4 servings

Bread, cereal, rice and pasta group
6-11 servings

The GIGO Factor
(Garbage In, Garbage Out)

The teen years are a time when the body works hard in many ways. Pediatricians tell us that the normal teenage body needs between 2,500 and 3,000 calories daily to support this special time of growth and development. What this means is that while a healthy diet is important to good health at every stage of life, it is especially important that teens have a good diet.

Food—Your Body's Energy Source

Food provides the body with nutrients it needs to regulate bodily functions, promote growth, repair body tissues and maintain energy. You have to fuel your body so it can do its job. There are some basics you must know about how food keeps your body functioning. If you can understand why your body depends on you to feed it healthy foods, you are more likely to make a point of nourishing it so it can do its job, rather than taking your body for granted. The following information is not intended to serve as your total resource guide on food and nutrition, but rather as a brief overview on how foods sustain your health. Please refer to the suggested reading section at the end of this book for more information. In addition, your parents, the school nurse, and other nutrition experts and health professionals can help you learn more on ways to fuel your body right.

The ABCs *of Nutrition*

There are *six* basic classes of nutrients: carbohydrates, fats, proteins, vitamins, minerals and water. In a nutshell, here's why and how they are important.

Carbohydrates. Carbohydrates are an excellent source of energy for the body, especially for your body's cells. Sugars and starches belong to this group. Fruits and vegetables, rich in essential vitamins and fiber as well as the antioxidant vitamins A and C, are good sources of sugar carbohydrates. Grains and whole-grain products, such as rice, cereals and breads, are good sources of starch carbohydrates.

Fats. Fats are necessary to supply our bodies with energy and are a part of the structure of our cells. Even so, many nutrition experts recommend that you limit your intake of fats. There are basically two kinds of fats: unsaturated fats and saturated fats. Unsaturated fats are those found in vegetable oils, nuts and seeds. These fats are better for you than are the saturated fats, which at room temperature are usually in solid form. Beef, pork, chicken and dairy products are high in saturated-fat content.

Proteins. The most basic and important role of proteins is building dense bones and strong muscles, and the growth and repair of the body's connective tissue. Milk, fish, dried beans, nuts, peanut butter, meat and soy products are all good sources of protein.

Vitamins. While the best way to get vitamins is to eat many different foods, some nutritionists recommend taking a daily multivitamin tablet as well. Check with your parents before you do. [See the chart on pages 83–84.]

Minerals. There are some twenty-four minerals essential for your good health. The chart at the end of this chapter [pages 85–86] shows the essential ones and their effects on the body. As with vitamins, minerals are found in a variety of foods. Multivitamins tablets also contain important minerals.

Water. The body needs water to function; it is essential to the body sustaining itself. Your body is 70–80 percent water with your brain and heart being 75 percent water, and your blood being 83 percent. Water is vital to all your body functions: circulatory, digestive, elimination and temperature control.

Don't neglect to fuel your body properly. If your body is not properly nourished, every system of your body can be harmed, and your ability to think well and to make other healthy choices about your life and your well-being can be impaired.

High-Power Foods for High-Power Performance

Ask any female athlete and she will tell you that during training and performing, she fuels her body completely differently than she does in the off-season. During the time she expects her body to "output" its best, she "inputs" the best. Even if you aren't an athlete, perhaps you've practiced this same principle. When you have a really big exam or semester finals, do you get to bed early and wake up to a good breakfast? If you feel a cold coming on, do you drink a lot of fluids, take vitamin C, and make sure you get the rest you need? If you're trying out for the tennis team, do you make sure you're well-rested the morning of tryouts, and that you've eaten a

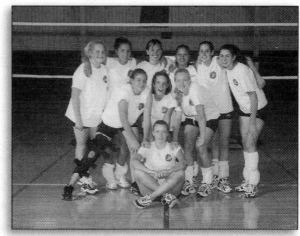

Fuel your body for high performance: Santa Fe Christian High School Girls Volleyball Team

nutritious, high-energy breakfast? Be that good to yourself all the time!

Why Parents Yell, "Eat Your Breakfast!"

If your mom and dad are like mine, you probably hear the words "Eat some breakfast!" on a daily basis. I liked hearing this line about as much as "Get your homework done." Since my taste buds didn't wake up until around 10:00 A.M., eating breakfast was even worse than having homework to do.

But Mom and Dad insisted for a good reason. Eating breakfast will help you have a better day. Yes, it really is that simple! When I eat breakfast, I am more likely to have my brain show up and help me out with tasks like thinking clearly—a function that can be very helpful in making good choices, in expressing myself and in doing well on all the things I need to do.

Eating Breakfast Is About Fueling the Brain

People who eat breakfast think more clearly, have more energy and are more creative in the morning than those who don't eat breakfast. This is because foods, especially fruits and grains, steadily release glucose, fueling the brain. Brain cells, like the rest of the body, require proper feeding in order to function correctly. Deprived of proper nutrients, the brain cannot perform at peak efficiency. How the brain functions so depends on how it is fueled that if you skip meals, it can't and won't function at its best.

3 X 3 = 6, Right?

It wasn't difficult to figure out that on those mornings when I didn't eat breakfast, I operated at a different level of efficiency than when I did eat breakfast. This was especially apparent on those days when I took an early morning test or quiz in one of my classes. I discovered that when I skipped breakfast, I'd frantically try to remember things, but the facts just didn't come to me—even though I had studied and knew the answers were safely tucked away in one of those little compartments in my brain. The problem was, without breakfast, I just couldn't seem to locate the little compartment that contained the answers. I just couldn't think as clearly. Sometimes I ended up completely bombing the test, like the morning of a big math quiz. I merrily sailed through the quiz thinking, "Gee, this is easy!"—all the while adding the numbers instead of multiplying them as the directions called for. Needless to say, I failed the quiz.

Not only could I not think as clearly without breakfast, but my energy level dragged. On top of that, I'd be cranky and tense and short with my friends—even my teachers. It wasn't until I finally realized that these things happened on those days when I skipped eating before I left home that I understood the best reason for eating breakfast.

A Pure Recipe for Eating Breakfast

If you're like most teens, the morning is a mad rush to get to school. Planning the night before can help to make breakfast time a little easier. If the breakfast table is set with the plates, bowls, glasses and silverware you and your family need, you will be more likely to eat something nutritious in the morning to get your day off to the right start. Eating just anything isn't good enough. For example, if you drink sodas in the morning, or eat too much sugar on your cereal, you are going to be really wired and hyper. And when the rush wears off, you are going to "crash"—to run out of energy.

For those days when you are running late, if you buy fruits and breakfast bars high in nutrients you can eat them on your way to school. The important thing is to eat those things that will nourish your growing body and sustain your day of activities. Remember the goal: Nourish your body; fuel your brain.

"It's Only 10:00 A.M. but I Gotta Have Food, Now!"

So you ate breakfast at seven o'clock, and it's only ten o'clock—but you're famished! Lunch is an hour and a half away. Chances are your body needs fuel! What's the solution? Food.

I recommend you pack extra snacks in a thermal lunch bag and keep them in your locker or backpack for these hungry times. If you have access to a cafeteria or snack dispenser that sells fruit, milk or juices, so much the better. The important thing is to eat what's good for you, food that will feed your growing body as well as provide energy to sustain your activities. You will actually feel an energy boost after eating these types of foods, instead of an energy drain that junk food can give you. For example, if you're on your way to your physical education class—a class which you've made a pact with your-self to get a good workout in—rather than grabbing a bag of cookies or chips from the dispenser, buy an energy bar or bag of nuts instead.

Choose foods that will not only quiet the hunger pangs but also provide energy.

Hungry Between Each and Every Class?

If your school doesn't have food-dispensing machines that carry energy- and nutrition-rich foods, or if you don't have the money to purchase dispenser snacks, then bring some from home. Veggie sticks (carrots and celery), nuts and seeds and fresh fruit are great pick-me-up boosts and are easy snacks to pack in your backpack or leave in your locker.

There are many high-energy snack foods you can buy and take to school. You can even make them. Here's my favorite one:

Energy Bars

Mix 1 cup all-natural peanut butter, $\frac{1}{3}$ cup nonfat dry milk, and 2 tablespoons of honey together until smooth and add any of the following: One cup of raisins, 2 tablespoons of chopped nuts or shredded coconut, $\frac{1}{3}$ cup of wheat germ or crushed whole grain cereal flakes. For a real treat, add chocolate chips. Roll into balls and store in a sealed plastic bag.

The 4:00 P.M. Pit-Stop: The Fridge

You've just arrived home from school, and the kitchen is your usual pit-stop on the way to your room. As always, you are famished. Even the carrot sticks in the refrigerator look good at this point, but you know you need something more substantial. Still, with dinner less than two hours away, and with lasagna—your most favorite food—being served, you want to show up at the family dinner table three-helpings hungry.

After school is a good time to eat more fresh fruits and vegetables. But you are *starving*. You can stave off the hunger pangs and still get an energy boost. A melted cheese sandwich, for example, is nutritious, and it will help you make it until dinner is served. And it's easy and quick to make. Simply toast two slices of whole grain bread. Put one or two slices of cheese on a sandwich. Microwave for thirty seconds.

Another solution is to make a tasty shake. Poor one cup of milk into the blender. Add two cups of fresh or frozen fruit—bananas, peaches and berries. Blend. You can even prepare the fruit ahead of time for these shakes and store them in the refrigerator.

Trying to wean yourself from stopping by the local convenience store so as to break the habit of eating low-nutrient junk food, but you love the taste of something sweet after school? Try filling plastic ice-pop molds with your favorite fruit juice and freezing the night before. Fruit pops are great fill-ins when your taste buds are screaming for something sweet.

Experiment a little. The goal is to find foods that are quick and easy to make as well as being a tasty means for you to eat nutritiously.

The 7:00 P.M. Craving Craze

It's a couple of hours after dinner, and you've still got hours of homework to do, but you're beginning to feel "brain dead." Once again, high-nutrient snacks are the key. If you're really talking about a couple of hours of homework, make yourself a fruit shake. Also good for boosting brainpower are foods like a hard-boiled egg, or fruits dipped in honey or yogurt.

Eat Like a Bird—All Day Long

My mother is the highest-energy person I've ever known. She also eats like a bird (and has maintained the same weight for nearly twenty-five years). But if you ask her how many times a day she eats, she'll reply, "I only eat once— all day long!"

Maybe that's her secret to high energy. Nutritionists report that it may be healthier to snack all day than to eat three large meals a day. Several smaller meals a day are actually easier on the body's overall functioning. This is because meals spread over the day help keep the body's blood sugar, or glucose, at a stable level. Because glucose is the primary source of energy in the body, it makes sense to maintain a steady level for greatest efficiency.

Get Food-Smart: Why Friends and Music Go Great with Meals

Here are a couple of other tips on making the most of fueling your body in the best ways possible.

- Relaxation goes great with food! If you're like most teens, life is a constant series of dashing from one place to the next, and you find yourself always in a hurry. Try to slow down when you're eating. When you consume food, your body needs to digest it. Allow your body to do its job.

- Music goes great with food! Nutritionists have learned that if you eat your food while listening to relaxing music (yes, that's the catch!), you'll eat slower. When listening to fast music you automatically tend to keep pace with its beat. Slowing down helps your body metabolize your food more efficiently. It also helps you digest your food and enjoy your meal more, so that you feel a greater sense of satisfaction when you're finished eating. This greater sense of satisfaction keeps you from wanting to snack again later on.

- Friends are a nice complement to dining. When eating in the cafeteria or at your favorite "hot spot," join friends. Being with your favorite friends can make dining enjoyable and a social experience. Again, the goal is to make mealtime a period of peace, relaxation and downtime. The same is true at home. Make a point of making mealtime a time to enjoy your food and the company of your family.

Fuel your body so it can stay in good health and sustain you in all that you ask of it. Start now. Nutritional savvy is something you can use your entire lifetime. The following charts and the next chapter will show you how.

Essential Vitamins

Vitamin		Good Sources	Main Functions	Effects of Deficiency	Effects of Overdose
FAT SOLUBLE	A	Liver; eggs; cheese; milk; yellow, orange, and dark green vegetables and fruit	Maintains healthy skin, bones, teeth, and hair; aids vision in dim light	Night blindness; rough skin; dry eyes; poor growth of bones and teeth	Blurred vision; headaches; fatigue; liver and nerve damage
	D	Milk; eggs; liver; exposure of skin to sunlight	Maintains the bones and teeth; helps in the use of calcium and phosphorus	Rickets in children (bones and teeth do not develop properly)	Calcium deposits in body; hearing loss
	E	Margarine; vegetable oils; wheat germ; whole grains; legumes; green, leafy vegetables	Aids in maintenance of red blood cells, vitamin A, and fats	Rupture of red blood cells	Unclear
	K	Green, leafy vegetables, potatoes; liver; made by intestinal bacteria	Aids in blood clotting	Hemorrhage; slow clotting of blood	Unclear
WATER SOLUBLE	B$_1$	Pork products; liver; whole-grain foods; legumes	Aids in carbohydrate use and nervous-system function	Beriberi (damage to nervous-system, heart, and muscles)	Unclear
	B$_2$ (Riboflavin)	Milk; eggs; meat; whole grains; dark green vegetables	Aids in metabolism of carbohydrates, proteins, and fats	Skin disorders; sensitive eyes	Unclear
	B$_3$ (Niacin)	Poultry; meat; fish; whole grains; nuts	Aids in energy metabolism	Pellagra (diarrhea, skin disorders, depression)	Ulcers; abnormal liver function
	B$_6$ (Pyroxidine)	Meats; poultry; fish; whole-grain foods; green vegetables	Aids in protein, fat, and carbohydrate metabolism	Skin disorders; anemia	Dependency; depression; irritability
	B$_{12}$ (Cobalamin)	Meat; fish; poultry; eggs; milk; cheese	Maintains healthy nervous system and red blood cells	Anemia; fatigue	Unclear

Essential Vitamins *(continued)*

Vitamin	Good Sources	Main Functions	Effects of Deficiency	Effects of Overdose
WATER SOLUBLE				
Folate	Green, leafy vegetables; legumes	Aids in formation of red blood cells and protein	Anemia; fatigue	Unclear
Pantothenic acid	Organ meats; poultry; fish; eggs; grains	Aids in energy metabolism	Vomiting; insomnia; fatigue	Diarrhea
Biotin	Organ meats; poultry; fish; eggs; peas; bananas; melons	Aids in energy metabolism	Abnormal heart function; skin disorders; loss of appetite	Unclear
C (Ascorbic acid)	Citrus fruits; green vegetables; melons; potatoes; tomatoes	Aids in bone, teeth and skin formation; resistance to infection; iron uptake	Scurvy (bleeding gums, loose teeth, wounds that do not heal)	Dependence; nausea; diarrhea

From Prentice Hall Health: Skills for Wellness by B. F. Pruitt, Kathy Teer Crumpler, and Deborah Prothrom-Stith. ©1997 by Prentice Hall. Used with permission.

Essential Minerals

Mineral	Good Sources	Main Functions	Effects of Deficiency	Effects of Overdose
Calcium	Milk and milk products; dark green, leafy vegetables; tofu; legumes	Helps build and maintain bones and teeth; nerve and muscle function; blood clotting	Rickets in children; osteoporosis in adults	Unclear
Phosphorus	Meat; eggs; poultry; fish; legumes; milk and milk products	Helps build and maintain bones and teeth; energy metabolism	Weakness; pain	Can create calcium deficiency
Magnesium	Leafy green vegetables; legumes; nuts; whole-grain foods	Helps build bones and protein; energy metabolism; muscle contraction	Weakness; mental disorders	Unclear
Sodium	Table salt; processed food; soy sauce	Helps maintain water balance; nerve function	Muscle cramps	Associated with high blood pressure
Chlorine	Table salt; soy sauce; processed foods	Helps maintain water balance; digestion	Growth failure; loss of appetite	Vomiting
Potassium	Vegetables, fruits, meat, poultry, fish	Helps maintain water balance and make protein; functioning of heart and nervous system	Muscular weakness; confusion; abnormal heart function	Muscular weakness; vomiting
Sulfur	Milk and milk products; meat; poultry; fish; legumes; nuts	Forms part of some amino acids and B vitamins	Unclear	Unclear
Iodine	Seafood; iodized salt	Helps in metabolism as part of thyroid hormone	Goiter (enlargement of thyroid); mental and physical retardation in infants	Abnormal thyroid function

Essential Minerals *(continued)*

Mineral	Good Sources	Main Functions	Effects of Deficiency	Effects of Overdose
Iron	Red meats; seafood; legumes; green, leafy vegetables; fortified cereals; dried fruits	Part of red blood cells; helps in energy metabolism	Anemia (weakness, paleness, shortness of breath)	Damage to liver and heart
Selenium	Seafoods; meats; organ meats	Helps break down harmful substances	Muscle weakness and pain; heart damage	Nausea; nerve damage; fatigue
Zinc	Meats; poultry; seafood; milk; whole-grain foods	Part of many substances that help carry out body processes	Slow growth rate in children; slow healing	Nausea; diarrhea
Fluorine	Fish; fluoridated water; animal foods	Helps form strong teeth and bones	Tooth decay	Discoloration of teeth

From Prentice Hall Health: Skills for Wellness by B. F. Pruitt, Kathy Teer Crumpler, and Deborah Prothrom-Stith. ©1997 by Prentice Hall. Used with permission.

8

"You Are What You Eat": Making Smart Choices About Food

*A woman's life can really
be a succession of lives, each revolving
around some emotionally compelling situation
or challenge, and each marked off by
some intense experience.*

—WALLIS, DUCHESS OF WINDSOR

"A Double Cheeseburger, French Fries and a Shake, Please!"

Marsha doesn't like to eat breakfast. Her friend, Elaine, doesn't eat breakfast on a regular basis either, though on occasion she will purchase a carton of juice and a Danish from the snack dispensing machine around mid-morning. At noon, the girls prefer to drive to the local fast food restaurant for lunch rather than eat in the school cafeteria. Each day they eat pretty much the same thing: a double cheeseburger, French fries and a strawberry shake. Sometimes they even have a double order of fries. After school, they join their friends for a snack of fast foods at a local mini-market. Does this sound like your eating habits?

Health experts say, "We are what we eat." Keeping this expression in mind, it's best to make smart choices about our food. As you learned in the last chapter, your body needs nutritious foods in order to regulate bodily functions, promote growth, repair body tissues and, of course, to get energy. But how do you know if having a bowl of soup is more nutritious than having pizza?

Pizza or Soup? How to Decide Which Is More Nutritious

When I was in junior high, my mother worked in a large office building just one block from my school. Every day after school I would go there. The instant I arrived at her office, I tossed my books in a chair and immediately headed for the office lunch room to raid it for something to eat. The lunch room was always stocked with an assortment of things such as fruit and packaged foods that were quick and easy to prepare. Sometimes I would have a piece of fruit, but mostly my taste buds went for the six-inch pizza that needed only to be zapped for three minutes in the microwave, or a cup of instant soup that I only needed to add water to and then microwave for a minute or two.

The pizza was my favorite!

How did I decide if I was going to have a pizza or a cup of soup? I based it on what seemed logical to me—at the time: If I was trying to "be good," I'd opt for the cup of soup. My reasoning was that a cup of soup was better for me and had fewer calories than the pizza did.

I was dead wrong about the nutrition value in both these foods. But I was right about calories being an important consideration—even if at the time I didn't know how to tell one calorie from another.

Watching What You Eat Means More than Just Keeping Your Eyes Open: Count Calories

A calorie is a unit of measurement—it's the amount of energy released when nutrients are burned by the body. A calorie is a calorie, whether you are talking about a calorie derived from a scoop of ice cream or from a stalk of celery.

The number of calories, as well as the nutritional value of the calorie, is important information. You see, I assumed that a cup of soup was much more wholesome for me than a pizza. I figured that by passing up a pizza I was exercising maximum willpower, and quite frankly, I was very happy with myself for doing that. In fact, each food had the same number of calories—but there were major differences in their food value. Whereas the pizza had 18 percent of the recommended daily maximums of fat, the soup had 20 percent. Whereas the pizza had 9 percent of the recommended daily maximums of sodium, the soup had a whopping 56 percent. Whereas the pizza had adequate amounts of protein and vitamins A and C, and adequate amounts of calcium and iron, the soup had not one trace of any protein, vitamins or minerals in it. And even though the pizza had 5 percent of the recommended daily maximums of cholesterol—whereas the soup had none—the pizza, overall, was still the better of the two foods! If only I had known then what I know now, I could have enjoyed the pizza without feeling like it was an unhealthy choice and known that it was better for me than the boring soup! Today, I make better choices about the calories I consume.

Here is some basic, but important, information on the almighty calorie.

1. Foods differ a great deal in calories. As you can also see from the Calorie Comparison inset that follows, a quarter-pound hamburger with cheese has about 550 calories, while 1 cup of cooked spaghetti with red sauce

has about 165. An apple has approximately 75 calories while one chocolate-chip cookie has 180.

Calorie Comparison

1 quarter-pound cheeseburger with a bun = 550; 1 cup of French fries = 650; 1 Coke = 150; 1 fudge sundae = 850; 1 slice of wheat bread = 65; 1 stalk of celery = 5; 1 cup of chocolate (whole) milk = 210; 1 cup of cooked spaghetti with red sauce =165; 1 slice of cheese pizza = 300; 1 medium size apple = 75; 1 orange = 60; 1 chocolate-chip cookie = 180.

2. The more calories a food has, the more energy it contains. If you compare the energy you would get from a cup of cooked spaghetti with the quarter-pound hamburger, you will see that the quarter-pound hamburger supplies your body with more energy than spaghetti. If you need the energy, like if you were fueling your body because you still had a long list of things to do, a hamburger, even though high in calories, might be a better choice than a cup of spaghetti.

3. The amount of weight you gain or lose depends less on the amount of food you eat than on the number of calories you consume. For example, one ten-ounce carton of French fries contains about 890 calories, while the same ten ounces of boiled potatoes has about 145 calories. Sometimes I hear someone say, "Oh, I'm not eating lunch (or dinner) because I'm trying to lose weight." Equating skipping a meal with weight loss can be

as misleading as equating how much you weigh with good health. Aside from not being good for the body, refraining from eating is not the only consideration in whether or not the amount of food you consume will show up on your bathroom scale. Earlier you learned that experts in nutrition have determined that teens need between 2,500 to 3,000 calories on a daily basis. Knowing the amount of calories you are consuming can help you figure out how to eat three to four meals each day with healthy snacks in between and still not gain unwanted weight.

4. The number of calories you consume is a deciding factor in how much you will need to exercise if your goal is to burn off weight before it's impossible to zip up your jeans. I'm pretty good about watching what I eat, but even so, there are certain times of the day when my willpower is zilch! It is at those times when I consume the most *calories.* Calories count. If you've eaten 6,000 calories each day for the last three weeks without doing much exercise, expect a weight gain. If you need to gain weight but you're taking in only 1,500 calories a day and running two miles each morning, expect a weight loss.

5. Some calories are better for you than others. It's not just the number of calories you consume, but the nutrition those calories supply. If you are trying to gain weight, a high-calorie food may be a good choice, as long as it provides useful nutrients. For example, a slice of pizza contains about 300 calories per serving, but it is unlikely that pizza alone will provide the necessary nutrients your body needs (unless it has been fortified with the necessary vitamins, minerals and so on). The same is true for eating a stalk of celery if your goal is not to put on weight. Even if you ate ten stalks of celery (5 calories per stalk) you may not gain weight, but again, it is unlikely that celery alone will provide the necessary nutrients your body needs to run efficiently.

How to Read a Food Label

So how do you make smart choices in foods? Read the label! It will help you decide if one food is better for you than another. Don't rely on an advertisement to give you this information. To judge the nutritional value of a food, read the label carefully. The Food and Drug Administration (FDA) requires packaged foods to be labeled with their ingredients, as well as with nutrition information. Here are the key questions to ask when reading a label:

- What are the ingredients? Are you allergic to any of them? Are they high in sugar or preservatives? Is the food high in sodium? What is the total fat content? Some nutrients are not good for you, such as too much fat or sodium. If the food is high in these, you may want to make a wiser choice of food.

- How many servings are in the container? A bag of potato chips may have twenty-five chips, but maybe the producer of the product is not suggesting that you eat them all at once and, instead, make them last for five servings, as is the case with the chocolate-dipped potato chips on the following page.

- How many calories are in one serving? Do the numbers of calories you are consuming make this item a smart choice?

- What are the percentages of valuable vitamins, minerals and other important nutrients? If the food contains them, great. If not, know that you aren't getting any (or enough) with this particular choice.

To Eat or Not to Eat: Putting Chocolate-Dipped Potato Chips to the Test

You're in seventh heaven—you've just discovered potato chips covered in chocolate—your two favorite foods combined into one! But as you're reaching for the bag, you wonder how nutritious this dream snack is. Everything you need to know is on the label.

First, recognize that one serving doesn't mean the entire bag, but, rather, just five chips! Five chips? Can anyone ever eat just *five chips?* The bag has five servings or twenty-five chips. Remember, each serving—only five chips—has a whopping 320 calories!

Do the math! One bag (it's easy just to keep munching and munching, mindlessly finishing the bag during a chat with your friends, or while you do your homework or watch your favorite TV show) has 320 calories multiplied by 5 servings (25 chips) for a grand total of 1,600 calories. Based on the recommended 3,000 calories per day, you've just eaten well over half a day's worth of calories!

Chocolate-Dipped Potato Chips	
NUTRITION FACTS	
Serving Size: 5 chips	
Servings per container = 5	
Calories per serving = 320	
Calories from Fat = 110	
% Daily Value	
Total Fat	42%
Polyunsaturated Fat	28%
Monounsaturated Fat	14%
Cholesterol	7%
Sodium	41%
Total Carbohydrates	10%
Dietary Fiber	4%
Sugars	26%
Protein	9%
Vitamin A	0%
Calcium	0%
Vitamin C	0%
Phosphorus	8%

What about nutrition? Again, refer to the label. As you can see, most of those calories come from *fat*. Yikes! And, there are almost no vitamins or protein, it's low in fiber, and has too much sodium. Is this a good snack? Hardly. Sorry. I absolutely love chocolate-dipped potato chips, too!

Making Smart Choices About Food

Why Skipping Meals Is a Bad Idea

Whenever I would try to tell myself that skipping breakfast would save me a few calories, it never really worked. For me, skipping meals only resulted in my adding more calories. I ended up defeating my own purpose, sabotaging myself. Though I tried to make it to lunch without eating anything, I usually found myself drawn to the machine that dispenses candies, chips and sodas. It doesn't take a genius to know that there are few, if any, nutritional benefits to these foods. For me, eating consistent meals throughout the day means I am more likely to resist the urge to spend my quarters on the machine dispensing calories. And besides, not all foods are high in calories. For example, for fewer than 200 calories, you can eat a bowl of cereal with skimmed milk and fruit and get a healthy boost of vitamins.

The Trick to Quieting a Screaming Taste Bud

Are your taste buds screaming for—well, what do they really want anyway? More food, or a certain food? If it's hunger, there are physical signs, such as hearing a growling stomach, feeling lightheaded, being irritable or having a headache. If you are hungry, eat.

Assuming that you have eaten a balanced meal but still your taste buds are *craving*—and you don't intend to appease them—here are some ideas on how to quiet cravings:

- **Drink water.** Sometimes you may feel like you're hungry when you're really thirsty. Water gives you a feeling of fullness. If you are trying to cut back on the quantities of food you are consuming, sipping water is also a good way to shrink your stomach so that you will desire less food. And of course, drinking adequate amounts of water also helps keep your skin healthy and is important to the health of your kidneys and liver, as well. Health experts say we need to drink at least eight 8-ounce glasses of water a day. If you're not used to doing so, at first it may seem difficult to drink so much water—especially since water has no taste. To get past the boredom of plain water, I add a flavor. Sometimes I put a slice of lemon in my glass of water; at other times I simply add a tablespoon of lemon-juice concentrate or a couple of tablespoons of my favorite juice. Personally, I like cranberry, cranapple and strawberry-banana blends, but add what you like. The goal is to drink the amount of water recommended by health experts.

- **Eat fruit.** Fruit is a good way to feed your craving without adding a lot of calories and can usually satisfy a sweet tooth. Most fruits contain vitamins essential for your body. Another treat that's comparatively low in calories and can take the edge off of a craving is a lollipop. But with any of these snacks it's important to remember—don't eat too many!

- **Add flavor and pizzazz to bland foods.** Eating healthy doesn't mean that food can't be tasty. Try picking up the taste with salsas and spices. Vegetables, baked potatoes, scrambled eggs and salads all taste great with salsa; and salsa has hardly any fat. Adding vinegar (it has zero calories) is a great way to increase flavor and liven up a salad, and it tastes great on vegetables, as well. Sprinkling olive oil on salads, vegetables and popcorn—rather than other oils or butter—can also cut fat and add flavor to your food. Air-popped popcorn tastes great sprinkled with spices, too. Try adding taco seasoning to your air-popped popcorn (a little goes a long way) to replace those nacho-cheese-flavored tortilla chips.

Be the Einstein of the Aisles: Shop Smart

Make a decision to shop smart. Chances are, with all of your activities, your parents do the bulk of grocery buying. Enlist their support in your desire to eat healthy. Talk it over with your parents and ask them to support your efforts to eat right by purchasing nutritional food, and less junk food—even when you beg for your favorite treats. And don't forget what a big help your friends can be. When my friend's brother needed to lose weight for wrestling, he and his buddies made a Pizza Pact, agreeing that they could eat only one pizza a week, and it had to be a veggie pizza. In addition, they declared their cafeteria table a TFZ: Taco-Free-Zone, banishing all tacos for one month. Randy told me later that he really wanted to stop at Taco Bell, but he worried that one of his friends would discover him. As he put it, "I'd never hear the end of it if I let the guys down."

Keep Healthy Snack Foods Around

If you keep healthy snack food around, they will be convenient when you are hungry. Bag up certain foods so that on your usual refrigerator run, you can grab the bags on your way to your room or out the door to meet your friends. Munching on cut veggies, pretzels, bagels and other low-fat snacks are a good way to satisfy your hunger while eating healthy foods. When you open the refrigerator you can see your daily allotment and have a better idea of the calories you are consuming.

Why Eating an <u>Entire</u> Pint of Ice Cream— in One Sitting—Can Be a Good Thing

Every once in a while it's a good idea to splurge and treat yourself to something you really love to eat—even though it's very high in calories! My thing was jelly beans. I would buy a bag of jelly beans and power them down! I mean, all at once! Then, I'd be so sick of jelly beans, and anything sweet, that I wouldn't want sweets for a long while.

I also loved ice cream! (I still do!) My mother had a habit of buying each member in our family a pint of his or her favorite ice cream. She did this each Saturday, her regular grocery-shopping day. The pint of ice cream was ours and ours alone! If we wanted to share it, fine. And if we didn't want to, that was fine, too. No one else was allowed to eat the other person's ice cream. Such were the rules in my house. But there was another rule, too.

"Jennifer," my mother would say, "this is your ice cream. You can eat it anytime you want. You can sit down and eat every bite all at once, or you can make it last until the next shopping day, which as you know, is at the end of the week."

I loved this rule, because every now and then, I would eat my entire pint of ice cream in one sitting. Not only did it taste just great to do that, but it also cured me of wanting any more ice cream until the next week! And, of course, sometimes I made mine last all week. And once, when my mother went out of the country for three long weeks, I nursed my pint of ice cream for twenty-one days! That was tough!

The point is, a system of treating yourself can actually help your long-term efforts to stop eating sweets on an everyday basis! When you know you will have a treat once in a while, you'll probably crave it less.

The goal is to get in the habit of making smart choices about what you eat.

Eating more nutritious foods and less fattening ones is a good habit, and one that serves us well for a lifetime.

Just as you make smart choices about food and your health, maybe you've decided your body doesn't need the weight it's carrying. The next chapter will help you make smart choices about what to do if you want to reduce your weight.

9

What You Should Know About Losing Weight

Healing is making whole,
restoring a state of perfection and
balance that has been lost.

—Andrew Weil, M.D.

Timber and Kitty

I have a friend, Karen, who is five feet, seven inches tall and weighs 112 pounds. My friend, Rianna is five feet even and also weighs 112. Whenever Rianna and Karen get together, invariably Rianna says, "I wish I were as skinny as you, Karen." Sometimes Rianna will even comment that she is "too fat." Is Karen underweight? Is Rianna overweight?

It depends.

I have two cats, Timber and Kitty. They are sisters, born the same day. I feed them the same food and show each of them equal affection. Though they are free to roam outside, both cats pretty much stay in the house. Just about everything about their lives is the same—but you would never know it to look at them. Timber is a most delicate little thing, while Kitty is a much larger cat. Despite their differences in body sizes, both are high-energy and very affectionate! Neither cat has ever been sick, nor does Timber have a tapeworm!

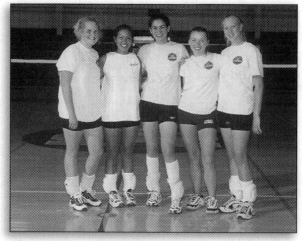

Classmates!

Six months ago when I took them for their annual health checkup, I asked the vet to explain why the cats were so different in body build. "That's just the way each one is built!" the vet explained. "Whereas Timber has a delicate bone structure, Kitty has a bigger frame."

The same thing is true for people. There is more than just a difference in height and weight between Karen and Rianna. As you can see in the photo of the girls above (all of whom are between the ages of fourteen and sixteen), bodies come in a variety of sizes and shapes.

Your "body type" is an important factor in how much you *should* weigh. (You'll learn more about this in chapter 14, "What Looks Best on *Your* Body?") We can't change the size of our bones. They are the supporting structures for the rest of our bodies, and all the dieting in the world won't make our bones diminish in size. Another important consideration is body composition—the amount of body fat compared to lean tissue, such as muscle and bone.

As for Karen and Rianna: At 112 pounds, is Rianna "fat"? No, 112 happens to be the "right" weight for her. Like my cat Kitty, Rianna has a large frame. In addition, she is an athlete, and some of her weight is in the form of muscle mass, not body fat. Karen is "perfect" for her body type, too. Contrary to Rianna's view of her friend, Karen is not skinny. In addition to being tall and "gangly," as Karen calls herself, she, like Timber, has a slight build—a delicate bone structure.

Rianna has full hips, whereas Karen has straight ones—shaped more like a boy's. No matter how much weight Rianna might lose, she will never change the shape of her hips. In jeans, she will never appear to have the straight lines Karen does. And as for Karen's complaint of wanting rounder hips (the reason she'd like to gain weight), it is unlikely that she'll get her wish of gaining weight only in her hips. Even when she gains weight, it's more apt to be distributed over her body, not changing her shape, but merely her weight. Just as a curvy teen isn't going to lose her hips by losing weight, Karen will not gain those curvy hips she's hoping for along with those extra pounds.

What Should _You_ Weigh?

Don't rely on the comments of your friends when it comes to deciding what you should weigh. If you are wondering what is the ideal weight for you, ask a health professional, such as the school nurse or your family doctor. And be realistic. Going on a diet may be good for your health, or it may have detrimental consequences. Dieting can take a toll on your body. The important thing is to get a medical opinion to help you determine if your body is ready to handle the demands of dieting. A health expert can help you design a plan that is best for you.

Following are some sensible ways you can manage your weight.

Smart Ways to Watch Your Weight

Don't Stop Eating

The first rule is don't skip meals. Skipping meals slows down your metabolism so that your body stores calories and burns them at a slower rate. This is especially true when you go on a crash diet. The body gets worried that it's going to run out of energy, so it starts to slow down to conserve energy and begins to pack away fat. Skipping meals is not only detrimental to your health, but it can actually cause you to gain weight.

Slowly Cut Back on How Much Food You Eat

Slowly cut back on the amount of food you consume at each meal. This will help you shrink your stomach. When you are in the habit of eating a big meal, the stomach doesn't feel satisfied unless it has the quantity. If you don't cut back in moderation, you can end up feeling tired and irritable. Cutting back means eating smaller portions, it doesn't mean cutting out foods altogether. A diet that robs your body of the essential nutrients, vitamins and minerals it needs to function properly can take a toll on your health and put your body at risk for health breakdowns.

As you begin cutting back, try using a smaller plate. Nutritionists tell me that by eating your meal from a smaller plate you trick the eye and brain into thinking that you have eaten a larger meal!

Avoid Fatty Foods as Much as You Can

If you cut out foods that are high in fat, you won't have to give up all of your favorite foods. How can you tell right off the bat if a food is fatty? Try rubbing it with a napkin. Is there a grease mark? If so, it probably has a lot of fat. To cut down on fat and calories, instead of regular dressings (usually high in fat), add yogurt, vinegar and other low-fat spreads and salad dressings to flavor your food.

Learn How to Make Tasty
Low-Calorie Foods

Watching your weight doesn't have to mean deprivation! You can watch your weight and still eat nutritiously—as well as eat deliciously! Take the time to find some tasty low-calorie recipes you can add to your weight-watching menu. Here are a few of my favorites:

Baked Pizza
Just 95 calories per serving!

1 large pita bread
4 tablespoons pasta sauce
4 tablespoons low-fat cottage
   cheese

¼ teaspoon dried oregano
½ teaspoon parmesan cheese

Split bread in half horizontally. Broil until toasted. Cover each half with sauce. Follow with cottage cheese. Sprinkle with oregano and parmesan cheese. Broil until cheese melts. Makes 2 servings.

Apple Nut Cookies

Just 75 calories each!

1½ cups rolled oats
1 teaspoon allspice
4 tablespoons shortening
3 tablespoons brown sugar

1 apple, cored and chopped
3 tablespoons walnuts
1 egg white

Preheat oven to 400°F. Mix together oats, allspice and shortening. Add sugar, apple, walnuts and egg white. Stir. Form 14 balls. Arrange on nonstick baking pan. Flatten slightly. Bake for 10 minutes. Makes 14 cookies.

Chicken Pasta Salad

Just 165 calories per serving!

3 cups chicken broth
1 pound boneless chicken
   breasts
2 cups of shell pasta
1 cup nonfat mayonnaise
1 teaspoon mustard
2 stalks of celery, thinly sliced

½ teaspoon celery salt
Ground pepper to taste
1 cup baby peas, cooked,
   drained and cooled
1 cup seedless red grapes,
   washed and cut in half

Bring broth to a simmer in medium saucepan. Add chicken breasts, and cook for 20 minutes. Remove breasts and chill. Cook pasta according to directions, drain and rinse in cold water. Mix together mayonnaise, mustard, celery, salt and pepper. Cut chicken into bite-sized pieces, and add to mixture. Add pasta, celery, peas and grapes. Toss together in medium bowl. Cover and refrigerate 1 hour. Makes 8 servings.

Potato Skins with Salsa

Just 49 calories per serving!

4 medium-size baking potatoes
Salt and pepper to taste
1 small tomato, chopped
½ cup black beans, drained
  and rinsed
2 tablespoons scallions

½ teaspoon ground cumin
½ cup shredded reduced-fat
  cheddar cheese
1 cup salsa
8-ounce container plain
  nonfat yogurt

Preheat oven to 450°F. Prick potatoes with a fork and bake until tender (about an hour). Cool 15 minutes. Quarter potatoes lengthwise. Scoop out flesh, leaving the shells intact. Place skins on baking sheet coated with cooking spray. Sprinkle with salt and pepper. Combine tomato, beans, scallions and cumin and then fill skins and top with cheese. Bake until cheese melts (about a minute). Top skins with salsa. Serve with yogurt. Makes 16 servings.

Drink Plenty of Water

Drinking water helps flush away toxins and fat, as well as curbing your appetite. Not only that, drinking cool water forces your body to speed up its metabolism to keep you warm. This helps burn calories. So, definitely drink your water!

Don't Eat Late at Night

Don't eat too late in the evening, and no late-night snacks unless it's vegetables. While asleep, your body isn't going to burn up those calories, nor quickly digest or metabolize that food.

Break the "Check It Out" Habit

Don't eat if you don't really need to eat. How many times do you open your refrigerator at home? I've read that the average teen opens his or her refrigerator about twenty-five times a day. Quite frankly, I think it's more than this. When my cousin's boyfriend visits her house, I think he opens it twenty-five times each hour! That's a lot of contact with food!

Here are some favorite tried and true ways to not consume food when you aren't really hungry:

- Tape a picture of yourself in your favorite swimsuit on the refrigerator. When I played sports in high school, be it a game day or just a long practice, I was simply starved all the time, and so I ate all the time. But I found that it was easier for me to burn off an extra helping of macaroni and cheese—and the candy bar—during a sports season than it was in the summer when I was mostly sunning on the beach with my friends and checking out the guys! So when I was between sports seasons, or during the summer, I'd tape a picture of myself wearing my favorite swimsuit on the refrigerator for incentive. The picture served as a reminder that if I wanted to be as lean and fit as I was during a sports season, then I needed to eat to nourish my body, but not eat just because there was food in sight. One look at myself in the photo and I knew that I shouldn't "pig out" or else I couldn't maintain my figure.

- Many teens tell me they are too self-conscious to put up a picture of themselves in swimwear on the refrigerator—especially if they have a bratty brother in the house, or if they have lots of friends over. So, instead, they put up a small mirror with a magnet on the back so that it attaches to the refrigerator door. This serves as a reminder to remember their goal to eating healthy.

- The pound-for-pound factor. One of my good friends, Sharece Hilton, used a technique she called the pound-for-pound factor. (I called it the "yuk factor.") As a reminder to herself to not eat when she really didn't need to, and most especially to avoid fattening foods, she kept a plastic bag filled with one pound of shortening (that's right, the white lard your grandmother uses to bake pies!) in the refrigerator where she could see it the moment she opened the door. Sharece said it made her think of what even a single pound of fat looked like, and since she found it repulsive, it instantly killed her desire to consume fattening foods.

Say "No" to Diet Pills

Under no circumstances should you take diet pills without the advice of your family doctor. As a matter of fact, do not start a diet or consume even over-the-counter drugs or health-food diet aids without getting professional and/or parental advice. Diet pills, especially those with caffeine, are bad for your heart.

Does Smoking Curb Your Appetite?

Perhaps you've heard that smoking can help curb your appetite. It's no secret smoking cigarettes is dangerous to your health. Aside from the fact that smoking puts your health at risk, the short-term effect of curbing your appetite is only temporary. Your body gets used to having nicotine and adjusts accordingly, and then smoking no longer works very well for curbing your appetite.

Is it true that people who quit smoking gain weight? Your metabolism will slow down some when your system is free of the nicotine—so if you are consuming the same amount of calories, you'll probably put on a few pounds—but this slowing is not permanent. Just like the curbed appetite and increased metabolism when you started smoking were temporary, so is the slowing of your metabolism and the increase in your appetite when you quit smoking. Again, your body will soon enough get used to not having nicotine and adjust accordingly. After this happens, the weight should come off naturally. You can usually count on this occurring from between six months to a year after you quit smoking. So if you get discouraged when you see the numbers on the scale start to climb, just remember it's only temporary! Even if you eat a low-calorie, low-fat diet you'll probably still experience some sort of weight gain, but just keep eating healthy and make certain to exercise. Adding some new aerobic activities, and doing them on a regular basis, can also help speed up your metabolism.

Burn Calories by Exercising

Taking in fewer calories is certainly one way to make sure you don't gain weight, but it's not enough. I am one of those people who gains weight by just

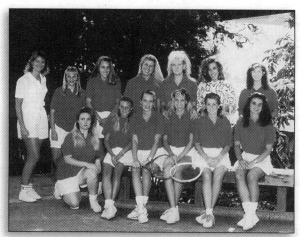

Participating in sports is a good way to burn calories.

looking across the room at a plate of desserts. In school, I was always most fit during the sports season. In the summer or off season, I gained weight. Now that I've been out of school for a couple of years, I've had seasons where I wasn't part of an organized sports team. During those times I really missed it as a way to keep my body fit and my weight down. The good news is that when I gain back the unwanted pounds, I revert back to that athlete in me. When I miss a season playing sports, I make certain to get involved in working out; I get myself to the workout center.

If you want to lose weight, you've got to get regular exercise. How long, how often and how hard you exercise will determine the amount of calories you burn. The simple fact is, the more muscles involved in an exercise, the more calories that are burned. (This is the reason so many people turn to sports like running, swimming, cycling, rowing, skiing, skating—these use a lot of large muscle groups.)

Walking two miles in thirty minutes burns 150 calories; drinking a soda can add 240 calories! The number of calories you burn depends on three factors: how long, how hard and how often you exercise. The best way to burn fat is to exercise long and slow (discussed in the exercise unit). When you exercise at slower speeds you body burns mostly fat (as opposed to carbohydrates or protein) to provide fuel for your muscles.

How to Fight Cellulite

Cellulite is a common problem for girls, some more than others. Having cellulite—those lumps that look like cottage cheese—doesn't necessarily mean you are "fat." Cellulite is pockets of toxins trapped in fat cells. It can form anywhere on your body, but it's most problematic on the thighs, abdomen and upper arms. Having cellulite is more a condition of how efficient your body is in breaking down toxins and carrying them away than it is a sign that you are overweight. This is why dieting rarely makes cellulite go away.

Even very thin women can have cellulite. Physicians say that cellulite is often inherited, meaning that some of us are more prone to it than others. The best way to combat cellulite is by eating a healthy diet, getting exercise and increasing the oxygen flow to the area affected by cellulite. Nutrition experts recommend a diet that is low-fat and low-salt, and high in raw vegetables and fresh fruits as well as drinking eight glasses of water daily (water helps flush toxins from the cells). In a nutshell, go easy on the carbonated sodas and processed foods.

Exercising regularly is another good way to fight cellulite, again because increasing the oxygen to the cells helps them purify themselves. You can also scrub the areas of cellulite with a loofah or bristle brush to increase the flow of blood (again, bringing oxygen) to the specific area affected by cellulite. Brushing in slow circular motions for two to three minutes each day when you are in the shower revs up your circulation and can help rid toxins trapped in cells. This will also make your skin appear more smooth and the cellulite less noticeable.

Looking Great, Feeling Great!

Try not to obsess too much over your weight. Keep in mind that the ideal weight for you may not be the ideal weight for someone else, and vice versa. Go for good health and high energy.

Another thing to consider is that sometimes firming, toning and building muscles is all you may need to look fit—all without the need to lose a single pound. Achieving that beautiful, fit look is what the following chapter is all about.

10

"Buffing Up" the Bod

*What we are all seeking is that
our life experience of being on the physical
plane will have resonance within our innermost
being and reality, so that we can actually
feel the rapture of being alive.*

—JOSEPH CAMPBELL

Exercise Your Right to Healthy Choices

Making "healthy choices" such as wearing the appropriate protective gear and clothing when you ride a bike, skateboard, Rollerblade or play contact sports; not using illegal drugs, including anabolic steroids; not smoking and avoiding smoke-filled areas; using a safety belt when riding in a car—all are ways of taking care of yourself. Making sure your heart, blood vessels, lungs and muscles work together to meet the body's needs is another. What's the best way to do this? By being physically fit.

Stimulating your muscles, bones, heart, lungs and blood vessels with regular exercise helps you attain and maintain—get and keep—physical fitness.

Xena the Warrior

In my school, there were the "regular guys," and then there were those boys who were really "buffed." We girls most often interpreted being fit as meaning we looked good. But having a body that is toned and taut is another degree of fitness.

A body that is toned—"buffed"—commands attention, and probably for more than the simple fact that a fit body is a beautiful body. A fit body indicates you value your body enough to take the time to get and stay in shape. There are lots of ways to do that; Marina's choice was body building.

Marina Carpenter went to my school in junior high, but she went on to a different high school than the one I attended. Still, she usually found time to hang out with my friends and me at least once in a while. Suddenly, after Christmas break our sophomore year, whether we asked her to go along with us to the mall or get together at one of our homes, Marina always seemed to have the same reply: "Thanks for asking me, but I can't. I'm going to the gym. But we'll do it another time for sure."

"Again?" we'd say, wondering how—or why—she wanted to spend so much time at a gym of all places. "Weight training," she replied. "I go every other day."

Weight training every other day sure seemed like a sacrifice—not to mention a lot of work—to the rest of us. "Marina, you don't look like you need to work out. Why are you doing all that?" my friend Jena asked. Marina shrugged and replied with certainty, "I want to have *great* muscles."

"You go, girl!" we replied. "Our own Xena the Warrior!" It wasn't that we didn't admire her efforts, it's just that school sports seemed enough of a workout for us. I played three sports. Besides living in a (sports) uniform, I found myself getting home at 7:30 almost every night. By the time I had dinner and got my homework done, I didn't get to bed until midnight. In addition to my athletics routine, I was enrolled in the mandatory physical education at school, so when it came to exercise, I couldn't imagine needing more of a workout than I was already getting. Most of my friends felt the same way. What we didn't know at the time was that exercise and fitness training are different. Very different. What Marina was doing was toning and building muscles through weight training. And it showed.

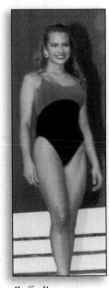

Buffed!

We might have thought Marina was taking it all too seriously that winter and spring, but when summer rolled around we were in for an eye-opener. We were at the beach one day, and it was clear that Marina's efforts had paid off. While we'd meant it when we said her shape seemed fine to begin with, after six months of regular body building it was spectacular! Xena the Warrior's body tone and developed muscles spoke for themselves—and it was obvious that everyone on the beach was listening!

An "A" for the Day—And for Life: Fifteen Minutes in Your Zone

Last summer I was trying to convince a good friend of mine to join me in playing for a women's softball team in my community. "No," she replied. "I hate sports, but I really do think it's admirable that you're as active as you are. I even envy you for enjoying athletic activities as much as you do, but it's just not my thing."

"Why do you have such a bad taste for physical activities?" I asked, knowing that every time I invited her to come with me when I worked out at a local workout center, she also declined. "Because," she replied, "I had my fill of boring exercise in high school. Really, for me it's about as much fun as watching grass grow."

It used to be that physical education had a bad reputation because it was so militaristic and boring. But things are changing in schools across the United States and I couldn't be more impressed—and supportive. There's a new P.E. in town, called, appropriately, New P.E.! Many schools now serve up a smorgasbord of lifestyle activities that include everything from fencing to indoor rock climbing.

Lifestyle activities are just part of the New P.E. To promote cardiovascular health, many schools have gone high-tech. Today, across the nation, each student in the class can be found wearing a heart monitor strapped to her chest with a watch on her wrist that displays her heartbeat. The goal is for each student to bring her body to the point of a cardiovascular workout and retain it for fifteen minutes. Students work at their own ability, working toward their goal to get themselves "in the zone." The monitor beeps when the student is above or below her target heart rate. Each student records how long she spends in her target zone, a range of beats-per-minute that is determined by age and weight. How does the student get graded? Fifteen minutes in your target zone is an A for the day.

So what if you're ten seconds off? Then you're ten seconds off an A! It's up to you—as most things are.

Exercise: The Billion Benefits of "Buffing Up"

While we all don't need to be Xena the Warrior like Marina was, we do need exercise. Look at some of the many benefits of exercise:

- Increases muscles strength and endurance
- Increases efficiency of heart and lungs
- Increases physical stamina
- Increases circulation
- Increases flexibility
- Keeps the heart healthy
- Adds oxygen to the body
- Improves digestion
- Relaxes nerves, balances emotions
- Increases resistance to disease
- Strengthens muscles, bones and ligaments
- Improves figure and complexion
- Helps reduce body fat
- Reduces risk of cardiovascular disease
- Improves posture and appearance
- Improves mental alertness
- Increases resistance to fatigue
- Improves self-confidence
- Increases social involvement
- Improves quality of sleep
- Increases ability to concentrate
- Improves self-image

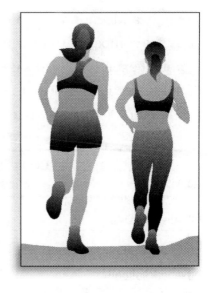

Pretty impressive list, don't you think? Make regular exercise a goal for life.

Punching the Remote Control Buttons Doesn't Count: Rating Workout Activities

Whether you work out in the gym, or are just normally active, your goal is *fitness*. Experts define fitness as cardiorespiratory endurance, muscular strength and endurance, flexibility, and body composition (the amount of body fat compared to lean tissue, such as muscle and bone).

Not all exercising offers the same benefits. In the chart below, the four areas of fitness are rated from 1 to 4 (1 = Low, 2 = Moderate, 3 = High, 4 = Very High) for different activities. Notice just how much they differ.

Activity	Cardiorespiratory Endurance	Muscular Strength	Muscular Endurance	Flexibility
Aerobic dancing	3–4	2	2	3
Ballet	3	2	2	4
Baseball/Softball	1	1	1	2
Basketball	3–4	1	2	2
Bicycling at 10 mph	3–4	2	3–4	1
Bowling	1	1	1	2
Calisthenics	3	3–4	3–4	3–4
Football	2–3	2	2	2
Gymnastics	1	4	3	4
Handball/Squash	3	2	3	2
Hiking (uphill)	3	1	2	2
Hockey	2–3	2	2	2
Jogging (6 mph)	3–4	1	3	2
Judo/Karate	1	2	1	3
Jumping Rope	3–4	1	3	2
Racquetball	3–4	1	3	2
Rowing	3–4	3	3	2

Activity	Cardiorespiratory Endurance	Muscular Strength	Muscular Endurance	Flexibility
Skating (ice, roller)	2-3	1	2–3	2
Skiing (cross-country)	4	2	3-4	2
Skiing (downhill)	3	2	2–3	2
Soccer	3	2	2	2
Swimming	4	2	3	2
Tennis/Badminton	2–3	1	2–3	2
Volleyball	2	1	2	2
Walking (brisk)	3	1	3	2
Weight training	1–2	4	3	2
Wrestling	3–4	2	3	3

From Prentice Hall Health: Skills for Wellness by B. F. Pruitt, Kathy Teer Crumpler, and Deborah Prothrom-Stith. ©1997 by Prentice Hall. Used with permission.

This chart can help you determine if you are already getting a great workout—or even if you are overworking your body. If you aren't sure one way or the other, check with your family doctor. You might also show this chart to your health education teacher or other expert in the field of fitness such as the fitness and training director at your local YWCA, workout center or family fitness center. Your goal is to see if your favorite way to exercise is meeting the needs of keeping you fit and in good health. [See colorplate 26.]

Are You Getting Enough Exercise?

When you were little, you probably loved taking frequent walks with your parents, bicycling to the park, swimming and playing for hours on end with

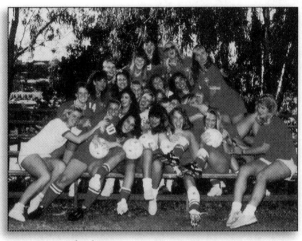

Exercise can be fun!

your friends. How about now—are you still as active?

Although you might feel like you're getting exercise because you are always busy running around with your friends, does the exercise you're getting now compare to the aerobic play activities of your younger years? Many teens assume that between their physical education classes at school, team sports and keeping up with the many activities in their lives, they are getting sufficient physical activity. But this might not always be true. In fact, too often teens do not get the proper amount of exercise required for good health. Experts tell us that today's teens are less fit than those just a decade before them.

If you feel that you need to do more to work on your fitness, perhaps it's time for you to get active again.

Before You Begin: A Word of Caution

If you aren't fit, work toward it. Regardless of what form of exercise you choose—be it jogging, an aerobics class or weight training—take precautions to prevent injury. Here are some important guidelines before you begin an exercise program. By following these easy precautions, you can help assure you gain in fitness safely:

1. Talk your plan over with your mom or dad, or your school nurse or family doctor or a health and fitness expert. This is especially important

if you are overweight, afflicted with any health problems, or in doubt about the status of your health. The reason for discussing it is to be sure you get on a plan that will benefit, rather than harm, your health.

2. Build fitness slowly, especially if you aren't in shape. Start off slowly and then pick up your pace and raise your expectations as your body adjusts to your regimen.

3. Eat nutritious, healthy foods. Remember the advice earlier in the unit about fueling the body for performance. Working out, while good for the body, also taxes it. Drink enough fluids before and after you exercise.

4. Always *stretch* before and after you work out to help avoid any muscle injuries. Warming up your muscles can prevent strains and tearing muscle tissue. Allow for periods of rest between strenuous exercising sets and sessions.

5. Make sure you're "belly breathing." We all know that our lives depend on air, on breathing! As strange as it may sound, many people don't know how to breathe properly. If you observe yourself and others, you may notice that breathing is often done with the chest, in short shallow breaths. This type of breathing (thoracic breathing) allows stale and unused air to be detained in the lungs. The healthy way to breathe is through diaphragmatic, or belly breathing. This is the way that babies and animals breathe.

Pay attention to your breathing. Make it a part of your workout warm-up. The goal is to breathe in deeply through your nose, expanding your diaphragm, and then exhale through your mouth. If you concentrate on your exhale, the inhale should come naturally. Before exercising, concentrate for ten inhalations and ten exhalations. This will help any stretching and exercising that you do afterward to flow smoothly, as it assists your mind in being like your body—alert and poised for action.

Finding Your M.A.T.E.
(Most Appropriate Training Exercise)

The best way to be healthy and fit is to make exercise a total part of your lifestyle. Exercise is the key. Many experts believe that the essential component of any fitness regime is that it be aerobic in nature. Aerobic means a level of activity that requires you to exert a good deal of effort, but doesn't consume oxygen faster than your heart and lungs can supply it. In keeping our bodies working efficiently and effectively on the inside, experts recommend three sessions of vigorous activity weekly, with each session lasting from twenty to thirty minutes.

Of course, there are any number of aerobic exercises and activities for you to choose from. There are gyms with everything from jazzercise to salsaerobics (a guided dance workout, choreographed to fast-paced salsa music). There's swimming, yoga, running, cycling and in-line skating (or Rollerblading)—to name just a few. If none of these options appeal to you, there's spinning, a workout done on a stationary bike; body sculpting or body pumping, which combine hand-held weights with body stretches, bends and steps; and kick-boxing and boxercising that will train you in self-defense, as well as give you a great workout. Experiment. Not everyone likes the same form of exercise. My friend Mia likes to go bicycling four afternoons a week, while my friend Kerry prefers a workout tape set to great music. By doing what you enjoy, you're more likely to stay with it. Following are a few suggestions for getting and staying fit, and to make exercise more fun.

Use the Team Theme: Think "School Sports"

My advice for teens is to join a sports team at your school. Here's why:
- **You'll be with your friends.** Being on a school team (you choose the

sport) is a great way to spend quality time with your friends. Being on a team can also help you win their respect and friendship. Many of my very best friendships came about from playing sports at school, both in junior high and high school. And the time I spent with my team members was a wonderful way to have fun, to laugh and shout and play—all great ways to release stress.

- **You'll get exercise on a regular basis.** For me, one of the biggest payoffs of playing sports was that I got to exercise on a regular basis. Most teams meet several times a week for practice sessions in prepa-

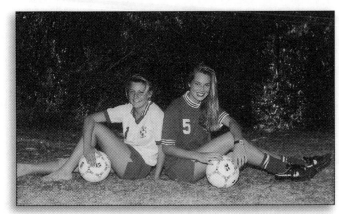

Sports, friends, fitness: great benefits!

ration for the day of the big game. A *regular* workout is exactly what the body needs to stay fit and healthy.

- **You'll get skills you can use for the rest of your life.** Being part of a team and receiving expert coaching is an ideal way to learn a sport, achieve proficiency at playing it and gain expert skills that you can use in many different areas for the rest of your life. While in junior high and high school, I learned to play tennis, softball and soccer. They are sports I loved then and now. I'm up for a game of tennis whenever I can work it in. Though my schedule doesn't allow me to play on the local women's soccer team, I do play on one of the three women's softball teams in my city. Because of the coaching and practice I received while in school, I can play these sports and do my best to help my team have a winning season. Moreover, I feel confident that I'm a valuable player. And the best part is that I have a lot of fun while staying in shape!

Boogie 'Til You're Buff: Go Dancing!

One way of exercising that most of us have a lot of fun doing is dancing. Whether you are doing the tango, salsaerobics or simply dancing to hip-hop, think of all the muscles you use when you dance—as well as all the calories you burn. A good fast-paced dance to music you love is very aerobic, and personally I find it good for the soul, too. If you want to make certain you get all your muscles involved, or feel like you'd like a little guidance, you can always use a workout tape that's set to the kind of music you like. This sort of workout is not only fun, it also provides you with some great practice for moves you'd like to perfect for school dances.

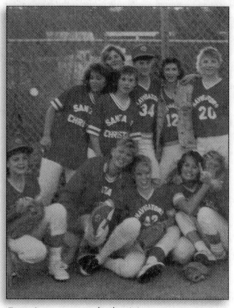

Exercise on a regular basis!

Take It in Stride: Power Walking

Even if you don't have an opportunity to join a sports team at your school or local YWCA, community center or family workout center, you can still exercise. One exercise almost everyone can incorporate into their regular activities is power walking. You'll need to walk at a brisk pace for thirty minutes at a time, at least three, if not five, times a week. When walking keep your upper body relaxed, with your shoulders eased down and back, your arms loose and low, and your fists unclenched. Even if you are overweight and have trouble with more strenuous workouts, you can begin walking and build up speed and stamina. If you are up to it, you might alternate between running two minutes and walking three minutes.

Kick It Up a Notch: "Challenge" Exercise

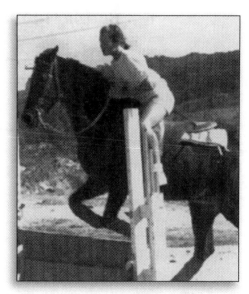

We all need to channel the desire for risk, adventure and challenge in a productive and positive way. Challenge exercise (CE) adds another dimension to the concept of physical fitness—the element of challenge. This challenge adds the bonus of mental well-being to the well-known euphoric experience of exercise, with a degree of well-being rarely experienced after a nonchallenging exercise. It is believed that it is this experience, rather than the fact that exercise is good for the body, that makes people return to CE sports.

Sorry, but cleaning out your closet with a friend doesn't qualify as CE (or aerobic)! Examples of CE sports are boxing, skiing, surfing, horseback riding, mountain and rock climbing, scuba diving, and other activities that combine a high degree of physical and mental coordination. (Non-CE sports are those such as calisthenics, jogging, walking or a game of golf with a motor cart.) And here's a bonus: Because of its benefits to both mind and body, CE provides an excellent means of "peak performance" and can even dramatically reduce stress.

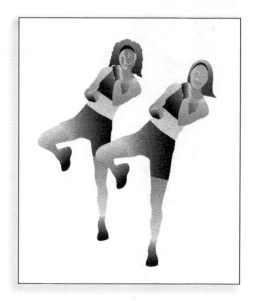

The Tendons Tug-o'-War: A "Stretch" Workout

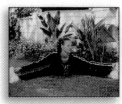
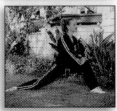
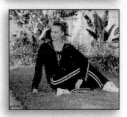

The beauty of a stretch workout is that it makes you feel energized as well as relaxed. Yesteryear the theme of exercise was "no pain, no gain." Today we have a kinder respect for our muscles. Stretching is now considered a viable form of exercise. It certainly is a balanced approach to overall fitness. Stretching tones your muscles as well as helps you to stay flexible. This is especially important so you don't injure muscles in your normal day-to-day activities. Have you ever been running, just playing a game of tag with a friend and, after only a short haul, felt a pain in the backs of your legs or in your ankles? It's because the muscles were not in the condition required for you to be exercising them as you were.

Stretching will give your body definition and make it toned and taut—without building muscle. Stretching exercises, like yoga for example, have a positive effect on your heart rate and metabolism; they also offer an added boost to your digestive system. Your local workout center, YWCA or community center often offers stretch-based exercise programs at affordable prices, but the nice thing about this activity is that you can do it at home and any time you want to. [See photos here and colorplates 46–56.]

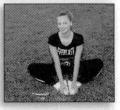
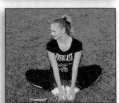
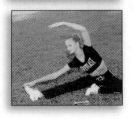

Need Extra Motivation to Exercise?

Would you rather have your wisdom teeth pulled than exercise? Here are some things that can add extra incentive to exercise regularly:

- **Sign a Contract:** Write down one fitness goal for the month. For example, "I want to be able to run (or power walk) one mile nonstop." Sign and date the contract and have it co-signed by a friend or family member. Hang it where you will see it daily.

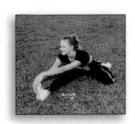

- **Set Up a Schedule:** Decide on a specific time and keep to this schedule. For example, you might exercise on Monday, Wednesday and Saturday between 4:30 and 5:15.

- **Record Your Results:** Post a chart on the mirror in your room for meeting your schedule as well as to record the results of how you're doing with your exercise goals.

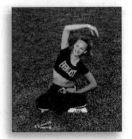

- **Reward Achievements:** When you reach a goal, reward yourself. Maybe you could buy a new CD or tickets to a concert you'd love to attend. However small or insignificant these may seem for all your efforts, they give you an incentive to look forward to, and serve as a measurement for meeting an important milestone: "I bought this CD for myself when I ran my first five-minute mile." Such "prizes" make meeting goals fun and memorable.

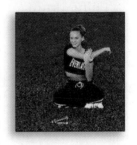

Prevention: Making Smart and Healthy Choices

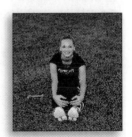

So far we've talked about choosing things that improve fitness. But making healthy choices also means choosing *not* to do self-destructive acts. Two of the most common are drinking

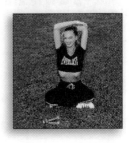

and smoking. When it comes to your health, be your own best friend. Don't worry that you won't be liked for making a choice to stay clean even if your friends or peers aren't. Keeping yourself drug and alcohol free is not only important to your health and wellness, but it is a good feeling and leads to self-confidence. Your body can count on you to do your part in staying healthy.

Beside the consequences of using substances, they have more side effects than you may think.

Friends Don't Let Friends Drink

Being drunk at a party is dangerous and shows a lack of self-worth. You've seen it for yourself. The other kids laugh at the person who is out of control. They may think it's amusing—but they aren't the ones slurring their words, staggering and acting in this embarrassing manner. But alcohol has even more serious consequences.

In addition to being illegal for teenagers to use, alcohol is a toxic drug that has many negative short- and long-term effects on your body. Upon reaching the brain, alcohol immediately has a depressant effect. In plain language, here's how drinking short-circuits your brain:

- It slows the speed of brain activities. Sometimes felt as "relaxing," what is being experienced is a loss of sensation and a decrease in sharpness of vision, hearing and other senses.
- Alcohol affects the part of the brain that controls muscle coordination, which is why someone may lose her balance or stumble.
- Alcohol depresses the part of the brain that controls breathing and heartbeat. Breathing rates, pulse rates and blood pressure, which initially increased, now decrease.

- The drinker may suffer blackouts, or loss of consciousness (even lapsing into a coma or death from alcohol poisoning).
- Alcohol slows response time in reacting, putting you at risk for accidents.
- With young women, alcohol also reduces inhibitions and has a high correlation to promiscuous behavior and date-rape cases.

Abstaining from alcohol is a healthy choice when it comes to your health and well-being.

Don't Send Your Health Up in Smoke

Another choice we make for our health is not to smoke. Let's face it. Smoking is not cool. And it is definitely not attractive. And of course, it's dangerous to your health, and can have deadly consequences.

The research is in: The U.S. surgeon general warning posted on the cigarette carton confirms that smoking causes lung cancer, emphysema and other illnesses. There are a lot of ways smoking takes its toll on your health: Smoking causes your blood vessels to constrict and this reduces blood flow throughout your body. The health of your skin and other body organs depends on blood flow to nourish them. By smoking, you are literally *starving* them to death. And, smoke damages the lungs. Your lungs and respiratory system carry oxygen to the bloodstream and remove carbon dioxide.

Aside from the fact that smoking puts your health at risk, it really is anything but glamorous. Most everyone other than another smoker finds it, well, quite frankly, disgusting. I can't tell you how many guys and girls I know who would like to go out with a special someone—"if only that person didn't smoke." Others said they didn't even consider dating someone who smoked for a number of reasons, including not wanting to be subjected to inhaling smoke—as well as "kissing someone who smokes is like *kissing an ashtray!*" Would you like to quit kissing, or quit smoking? No decision there! And though many teens initially start smoking because they thought it looked sexy, nearly every smoker I know says she wishes she had not started.

Aside from all of the health risks and negative appeal, smoking comes at the cost of countless beauty disasters. You'll smell of smoke—your hair, your hands, your clothes and your breath will all reek of it—which is a real negative when it comes to any sort of sex appeal. You'll also be tainting the beauty of your smile as you stain your teeth with nicotine. Even your fingers where you hold the cigarette can become stained a telltale, unattractive yellow. And it's terrible for the health of your skin. Because smoking starves your body of nutrients, water and oxygen, the result is dehydration, leaving your skin dry and pasty looking. Smoking also speeds up facial wrinkles.

If all this knowledge and advice is a little late in reaching you because you've already taken up smoking, now is the best time to quit. If you smoke, here are some helpful hints to help you kick the habit.

Butt Out: Tips on How to Stop Smoking

- Try chewing sugarless gum or sucking sugarless mints when a craving hits.
- Some people like to suck on lollipops because they last about the same length of time as a cigarette, and you can play with the stick when you have it in your mouth, so it slowly weans you from the hand-to-mouth habit that smoking involves.
- Use creative visualization to see yourself as a healthy nonsmoker and use

self-talk to counter destructive "smoking thoughts." When the craving strikes and you find yourself reaching for a cigarette, rather than saying, "I really want a cigarette," tell yourself, "I don't smoke anymore." Then focus on all the positive gains, like your clearer complexion, fresh new smoke-free smell, and standing among your favorite friends without having to worry that you smell unappealing.

- Let others know about your decision to quit smoking, but avoid constantly talking about it. Dwelling upon it will only serve to keep you missing the habit. Get support from your family and those friends who do not smoke. Keep in mind that there are support groups available in most communities. You can find out where these are by calling your local American Cancer Society chapter. Also, your school nurse or family doctor will know. The suggested reading section at the back of this book also offers books that detail other ways to support your nonsmoking health habits.

- Many teens tell me they've had success in quitting with the support of a friend who wants to quit, too. There's nothing like a good friend to help you stay with your decision to stop smoking. Some teens also tell me that they challenge a parent to stop smoking and, together, support one another. Once you tell other people about your decision, stick to it. It takes time to break a habit, but be strong. You can do it!

- It'll go so much easier for you if you don't tease yourself with a few puffs or "just one" cigarette here or there. It just prolongs and encourages the obsession and the power of the addictive factors of the habit. But if you do slip and have a few puffs, or even a whole cigarette, don't use your slip as an excuse to give up altogether. There's always the next cigarette— the one that you don't touch—and the next day, when you don't smoke a single drag. Every day and every cigarette that you don't smoke brings you that much closer to being free of the habit forever. One of my good friends, Lisa, smoked. I tried everything to help her quit, but to no avail.

Finally, when she made up her own mind to quit, she made a plan and stuck to it. I was proud of her because I know how difficult it was for her. Though it wasn't easy, it wasn't impossible.

- Be proud of your accomplishment and reward yourself! Keep track of the money you would've spent on cigarettes in a jar or container. Once you've saved up enough, buy yourself something special or fun that you really want, maybe a new CD or a new item of clothing or a pair of shoes. An even better idea is to spend it on some activity that's not only fun for you but that also helps you stay fit (like a membership at the workout center).

- If you always like to have a cigarette when you're hanging around in certain places with certain friends who smoke, avoid those places and even those friends—at least during the first few days and weeks after you quit.

- Try a smoking aid to help you quit smoking. The "patch" is a small nicotine-containing adhesive that allows a steady, controlled level of nicotine to pass through your skin and into your body. The patch works by reducing your dependence on nicotine gradually. In some states, it is illegal to buy a patch without a prescription from your doctor until you are eighteen years old. In other states, you can buy the patch over the counter in a drugstore. Either way, they are expensive.

- Almost all brands of the patch suggest using a personal custom-tailored plan to help you break your psychological addiction to smoking. Used along with the patch, both can help you stop your dependence on nicotine. See your doctor or ask your parents or a trusted adult to help you decide which is best for you, and to help you monitor how safe it is for you.

    A word of caution: Read the labels on these and other drugs to control substance abuse very carefully. The patch—as is true of most aids to help you control and stop smoking—is designed to release different doses of nicotine into your bloodstream. If you have been smoking up to seven cigarettes a day, for example, but purchase a quitting aid designed for those smoking up to two or more packs a day, you can actually overdose on the nicotine that will be released into your bloodstream. This is another reason why, if you smoke, you should ask your parents to help you stop. Don't worry that they will be upset to discover that you smoke. Chances are, they already know. And if they don't, they will probably be happy to help someone they love break a habit that is life-threatening—as smoking is.

- Support antismoking laws and measures to keep restaurants and office smoke-free. Smoking is a real health risk, and helping citizens reduce their dependency on nicotine is a community concern.

Safe Choices About Safe Sex

The National Campaign to Prevent Teen Pregnancy reports that half of all first teen pregnancies happen in the first six months of sexual activity. Don't be naive about chances of getting pregnant if you aren't practicing safe sex. It only takes one time to get pregnant, or to contract a sexually transmitted infection (STI). Either choose not to have sex at all, or use contraception carefully *every* time. If you are pregnant, turn to your parents, a school nurse or a women's clinic to help you. Pregnancy is a huge life-changing event. Don't be pregnant alone, and don't think all you need is to talk it over with a good friend your own age. Teen pregnancy, whether you end the pregnancy or have your baby, is a decision that will affect many people's lives. Reach out and get the assistance you need. After all, even if in the beginning only you and the baby's father know about it, everyone will know sooner or later if you continue your pregnancy. Think for yourself and make smart choices about your own well-being. If you are pregnant or suspect you are, make smart choices about you and your baby's well-being.

Take Good Care of Yourself!

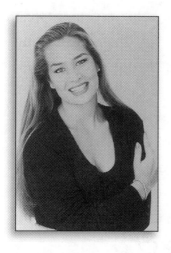

Health and fitness are important goals. Even though a challenge, reaching those goals can be fun—and they are certainly worth the discipline and hard work you put into achieving them. The more you practice healthy habits of working toward fitness and wellness, the more they become second nature, a lifestyle. And that's your goal.

As you'll see in the next chapter, rest, sleep and relaxation are also an important factors in your good health.

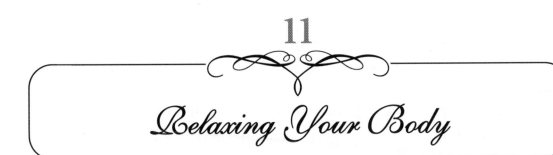

11

Relaxing Your Body

Meditation is to be aware of what is going on—
in our bodies, our feelings, our minds and the world.
Don't think you have to be solemn to meditate.
To meditate well, you have to smile a lot.

—THICH NHAT HANH

Sleep: Your Most Laid-Back Fitness Routine

Sleep, like nutrition, affects your level of fitness. Sleep is vital for good health. *Sleep is your body's recovery period.* During sleep your muscles relax, your breathing and heart rates decrease and your body temperature drops slightly. You've probably noticed a certain pattern to your body's ability to meet the demands of your life on a daily basis. For example, you probably wake up about the same time, get hungry around the same times each day, and get tired pretty much about the same time each evening. We call this twenty-four-hour cycle of energy flow (experts call these "behavior patterns") the *circadian rhythm*. Even your temperature, mood and alertness tend to rise and fall at roughly the same time every day. In other words, your body likes a predictable routine—such as going to bed at the same time each night, or having lunch at the same time each day.

How much sleep is enough? Health experts say that teens need between eight and twelve hours of sleep to maintain this intense stage of growth and development.

But not all sleep is the same. There are actually two different types of sleep: nonrapid eye movement (NREM) and rapid eye movement (REM). This sounds complicated, but it really isn't. In REM, which makes up about 25 percent of your sleeping time, the brain is still at a high level of brain activity. This is the stage of sleep in which you dream. In NREM, the "best sleep," your eyes move very little and your body reaches its state of deepest relaxation. NREM has four stages, each stage taking the body into a deeper and deeper phase of sleep, the last of these phases offering the body its best rest (primarily because the muscles in your entire body are most relaxed). Again, because we are so active, and because it is during a state of deep relaxation that the body renews itself, the NREM stage of sleep is very important to the health of the body. Fitness experts tell us that people who exercise regularly and are in a relaxed state upon going to bed spend more time in the NREM state of sleep than those who don't exercise.

Tips for a Good Night's Sleep

Here are some things you can do to get a restful night's sleep:

- Make sure you are getting adequate exercise. There is nothing like the rest that comes from the body's being tired and wanting to rest itself.
- Go to bed at the same time every night. The body likes a routine, one it can count on.

- Don't play heavy metal or music with a fast tempo. This music will rev you up. Save it for the morning or after school when your goal is to reenergize.

- Use mellow music to put you in the mood to sleep. This helps clear your mind of your schedule and hectic day. As you are listening, think about a positive and bright spot in your day. Let it fill your mind with uplifting, pleasant and reassuring thoughts as you wind down your day, and prepare to get the rest you need to have a great tomorrow.

- Don't eat right before bedtime. Your don't want your body to have to work at digesting food when you are trying to shut down for the night.

- Avoid stimulants such as caffeine and nicotine. These will keep you awake.

- Create a pleasant place to "snuggle in" and sleep. Choose soothing colors for your walls, decorate with your favorite pictures and snapshots of family and friends and your favorite stuffed animals.

- Don't make phone calls to best friends and boyfriends just before you crawl into bed. I know you are going to say, "What?" but trust me, there's a reason. Best friends and boyfriends get your mind going in a million different directions. When you're trying to shut down for the day, unless you are absolutely on mellow terms with these important people in your life, speaking with them very late at night will only cause you to lie awake for hours thinking about them. If you do that, tomorrow you'll be the groggy one with the puffy little eyes! Remember the goal: Allow your body to get to the NREM state as soon as possible.

Respiration Aspirations: Learn to Breathe Properly

In chapter 10, "'Buffing Up' the Bod," I discussed the importance of "belly breathing" in exercise. Belly breathing is also a useful tool for relaxing your body. Think about the last time you sat back, stretched and sighed deeply. In doing so, you completely filled your lungs and diaphragm with air and then let it all out slowly. This is your body's natural way of breathing. Here are the basic principles:

INHALE deeply, first filling the diaphragm area with air (stomach goes out). Continue inhaling as the lower part of the chest expands. Finish inhaling as the upper ribs are expanded and the top of the lungs fill with air.

EXHALE slowly. The air flows out smoothly from the top of the chest, down through the middle, and completely out as the stomach draws in.

REST for a few seconds. Begin the process again by inhaling deeply.

The following exercise is designed to help you relax through proper breathing techniques. To begin, find a quiet, peaceful place where there are no distractions. Lie down on your bed or on the floor. Get as comfortable as possible. Loosen any tight-fitting clothing. If your shoes feel tight, you may wish to take them off. Move your arms and legs around to make your muscles loose. Then, follow these steps:

1. Close your eyes.
2. Place your hands very lightly on your abdomen just below the navel with your fingertips touching.
3. Take a deep breath in and count slowly: one . . . two . . . three . . . four. As you inhale through your nose, your abdomen should swell out. This may feel a bit awkward at first if you are used to more shallow chest breathing. You may have to make a conscious effort to push your stomach. An alternative method for checking to see whether you are using your diaphragm appropriately is to make a "bridge" by placing a notebook on your abdomen. When you inhale, you should see the lower end of the bridge tilting higher.

4. After inhaling deeply, begin to exhale through the nose. Let the air out very slowly, counting one . . . two . . . three . . . four. Draw in the stomach so that your fingertips come together again. If necessary, make a conscious effort to pull in the stomach slightly.

5. Breathe in deeply: one . . . two . . . three . . . four.

6. Let the air out slowly: one . . . two . . . three . . . four.

7. Repeat this five more times.

8. Open your eyes.

Practice breathing this way as you lie in bed in the morning and again just before you fall asleep. This way you will get into the habit of breathing correctly.

In Tune with Your Body: Relaxation Through Music

Have you ever put on one of your favorite CDs and then found yourself dancing around the room? I have. And whenever I listen to my favorite tunes, and most especially when I end up dancing to them, I always feel an extra burst of energy—and it's the kind of energy that's free of all tension. It's a vibrant but calm and joyful feeling.

Just as music has the power to change your energy level, it has the power to change your mood. Perhaps you've brought yourself close to tears with a sad song or smiled over a happy one. Sound has a powerful influence over the way you feel. The work of numerous researchers has proven that whether you hear a sound consciously or unconsciously, your body hears the vibration and responds to it at the cellular level. While some sounds can keep you well and "in tune" with yourself, others create stress and can literally make you sick. The research of Dr. Sheldon Deal, a nationally known chiropractor and

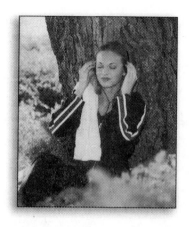 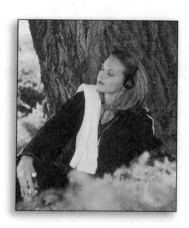

author, shows that loud and harsh sounds have a definite weakening effect on muscle strength. Over 90 percent of persons tested on an instrument designed to measure the effect of noise on muscle strength, called the electronic strain gauge, register an instant loss of two-thirds of their normal muscle strength while listening to loud and harsh sounds.

Let Music Put You in the Right Mood

It's good news and bad news that sound has such a powerful effect on us. So, we must use it to our advantage. For example, it's not a good idea to play music that has a fast tempo right before going to bed. Because it is stimulating, it has the opposite effect you want. When getting ready for bed, put on subtle, soothing and relaxing sounds. If the songs won't drive you crazy, mellow records from your folks' Old Fogies collection would work. The goal is to relax so you can get to sleep. When the body has been lulled to sleep by soothing music, you'll wake up in the morning feeling well rested. In the morning when you begin getting ready for the day, put on music that will put you in a positive and upbeat mood. This will help you feel jazzed and ready for the day at hand.

Reducing Brain Strain: Mental Relaxation

Relaxing your mind is just as important as relaxing your body. Visual imagery, sometimes called "visualization," is a powerful technique to produce positive, relaxing images and thoughts. Mental imagery is a little like a daydream. You may want to start by trying to visualize a pleasant scene, perhaps one you have seen many times. Try to reexperience the scene in every way you can, including the use of images from your senses—such as smell (for example, the scent of flowers), touch (the feel of the grass beneath your feet), sound (the sound of birds singing in the trees), and taste (the salt air at the beach). Soothing music may create a calm state and can also be used along with this exercise.

Be patient with yourself as you begin to learn mental relaxation. Don't get too concerned if at first your mind wanders off to other places. Simply redirect your thoughts.

To prepare, find a quiet place without distractions. Sit or lie down. Get comfortable. Loosen any tight-fitting clothing. Then follow these steps:

1. Close your eyes.
2. Take a deep breath. Imagine breathing in the clean air. As you breathe out, feel the relaxation spread over your body. As you take another breath, feel yourself floating down.
3. Tense and relax your muscles.
4. Imagine or picture yourself doing something relaxing. Get the full picture in your mind (some ideas for this are listed in the next section).
5. When you are finished, stretch your arms, take a deep breath and open your eyes.

Mental Maps: Exercises for Using Guided Visual Imagery

Here are some ideas for guided visual imagery:

- You are lying under the sun on the warm beach. The sand feels nice and soft underneath you. You're very calm and relaxed, almost falling asleep. The ocean breeze feels good against your skin. You can taste the salt air on your lips. You can hear the waves rolling in gently. You feel very comfortable, relaxed, peaceful, and calm. . . .
- You are walking slowly through a beautiful green forest. The only sounds you can hear are the sounds of the birds in the distance and of water flowing over a waterfall. It is very peaceful, and you continue to walk slowly and quietly, enjoying the calm and peacefulness. It is a warm day, but the forest is very comfortable. You have the forest all to yourself with nothing to disturb you. You begin to hum your favorite tune. . . .
- It is a lazy Saturday morning, everyone else is still asleep. A cool rain is falling outside, making gentle sounds that can be heard against your window. You are still sleepy. The fluffy covers on your bed are warm and soft. You bask in the thought of not having to get up, and you turn over and begin to daydream about something you like. . . .

Where Do You Want to Go? Creating Your Own Visualization

Using your imagination, create your own relaxing picture.

1. Think of a beautiful and relaxed setting that makes you feel relaxed.
2. Put yourself there and mentally describe what you are doing.
3. What's the weather like there?

4. How do you feel when you are there?

5. Why would you like to return to this place?

Visual imagery can be used for tasks other than relaxing. As you see your-self in conflict over a problem situation, try to imagine yourself dealing successfully with the situation. When you think about your thoughts, you have a better chance to be in charge of your emotions, and you are more likely to be in control of your behavior.

Progressive Muscle Relaxation

When you are nervous, upset or stressed, your muscles tense and tighten, especially the muscle groups around the head, face, neck and shoulders. Physical exercise and learning techniques to relax help you get rid of muscle tension and feel back in control. A great way to relieve stress and tension is to use a technique referred to as *progressive muscle relaxation*, a method in which you first tense a muscle (or muscle group), hold the tension for a count of five, and then relax the muscle. For example, if you wanted to relax shoulder tension, you would shrug your (right or left) shoulder up and try to touch your ear, and then hold the tension for a count of five. Then, you would relax it. When you do this, you can literally feel the tension draining away. Be sure to check out the suggested reading section at the back of this book for other ways to relax, and to learn specific skills you can use when you need them.

Now That You're Calm and Cool . . .

With your body healthy, fit and well-nourished, with your muscles and mind toned and relaxed, you've assured yourself a great advantage when it comes to looking beautiful. In the following unit, you'll learn how to dress to further enhance that appearance of beauty.

PART TWO

Health & Beauty: The Outside View

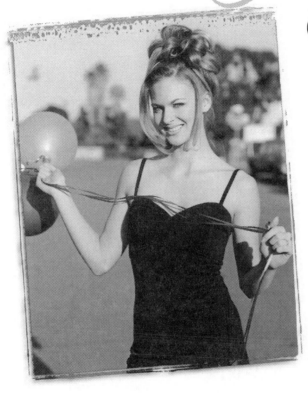

Beauty is in
the eye of the
beholder.

—Lord Byron

SPRING

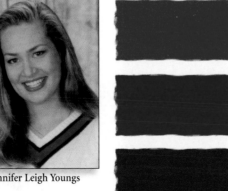

Tawny Flippen

WARM COLORS

SUMMER

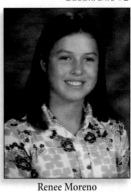

Renee Moreno

WARM COLORS

AUTUMN

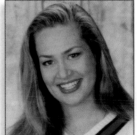

Jennifer Leigh Youngs

WARM COLORS

WINTER

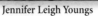

Lena Arcero

WARM COLORS

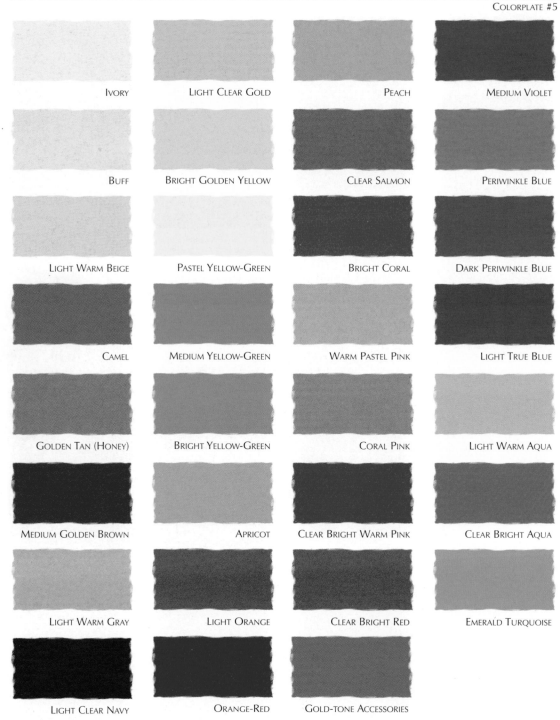

IVORY	LIGHT CLEAR GOLD	PEACH	MEDIUM VIOLET
BUFF	BRIGHT GOLDEN YELLOW	CLEAR SALMON	PERIWINKLE BLUE
LIGHT WARM BEIGE	PASTEL YELLOW-GREEN	BRIGHT CORAL	DARK PERIWINKLE BLUE
CAMEL	MEDIUM YELLOW-GREEN	WARM PASTEL PINK	LIGHT TRUE BLUE
GOLDEN TAN (HONEY)	BRIGHT YELLOW-GREEN	CORAL PINK	LIGHT WARM AQUA
MEDIUM GOLDEN BROWN	APRICOT	CLEAR BRIGHT WARM PINK	CLEAR BRIGHT AQUA
LIGHT WARM GRAY	LIGHT ORANGE	CLEAR BRIGHT RED	EMERALD TURQUOISE
LIGHT CLEAR NAVY	ORANGE-RED	GOLD-TONE ACCESSORIES	

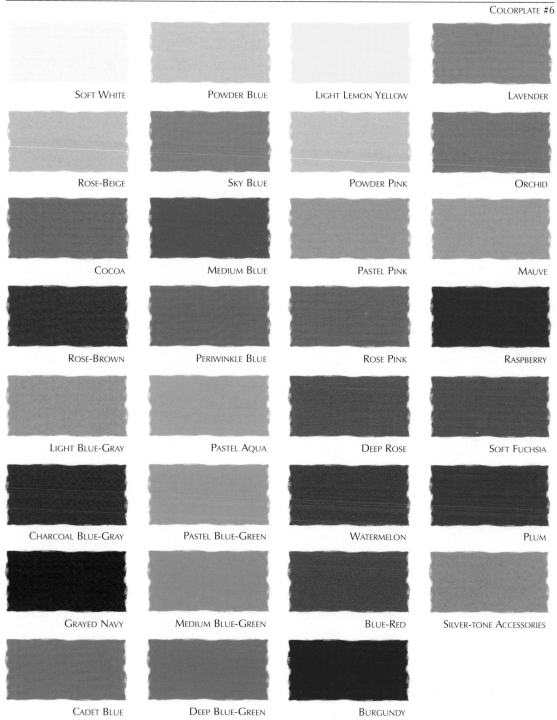

SOFT WHITE

POWDER BLUE

LIGHT LEMON YELLOW

LAVENDER

ROSE-BEIGE

SKY BLUE

POWDER PINK

ORCHID

COCOA

MEDIUM BLUE

PASTEL PINK

MAUVE

ROSE-BROWN

PERIWINKLE BLUE

ROSE PINK

RASPBERRY

LIGHT BLUE-GRAY

PASTEL AQUA

DEEP ROSE

SOFT FUCHSIA

CHARCOAL BLUE-GRAY

PASTEL BLUE-GREEN

WATERMELON

PLUM

GRAYED NAVY

MEDIUM BLUE-GREEN

BLUE-RED

SILVER-TONE ACCESSORIES

CADET BLUE

DEEP BLUE-GREEN

BURGUNDY

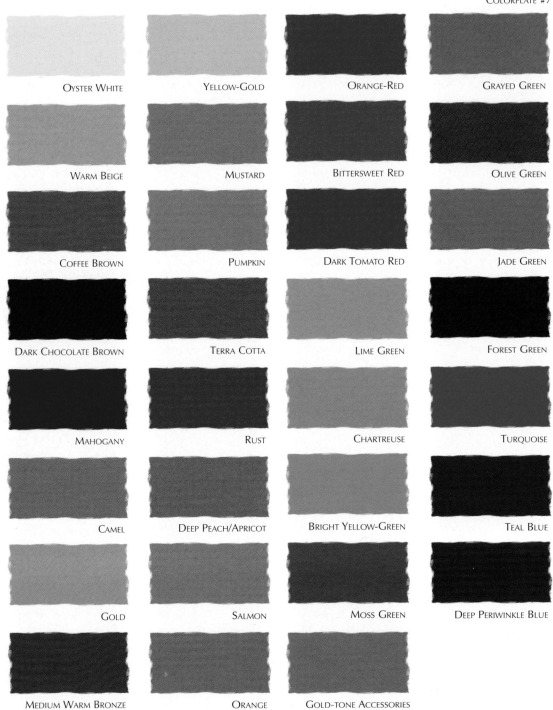

OYSTER WHITE	YELLOW-GOLD	ORANGE-RED	GRAYED GREEN
WARM BEIGE	MUSTARD	BITTERSWEET RED	OLIVE GREEN
COFFEE BROWN	PUMPKIN	DARK TOMATO RED	JADE GREEN
DARK CHOCOLATE BROWN	TERRA COTTA	LIME GREEN	FOREST GREEN
MAHOGANY	RUST	CHARTREUSE	TURQUOISE
CAMEL	DEEP PEACH/APRICOT	BRIGHT YELLOW-GREEN	TEAL BLUE
GOLD	SALMON	MOSS GREEN	DEEP PERIWINKLE BLUE
MEDIUM WARM BRONZE	ORANGE	GOLD-TONE ACCESSORIES	

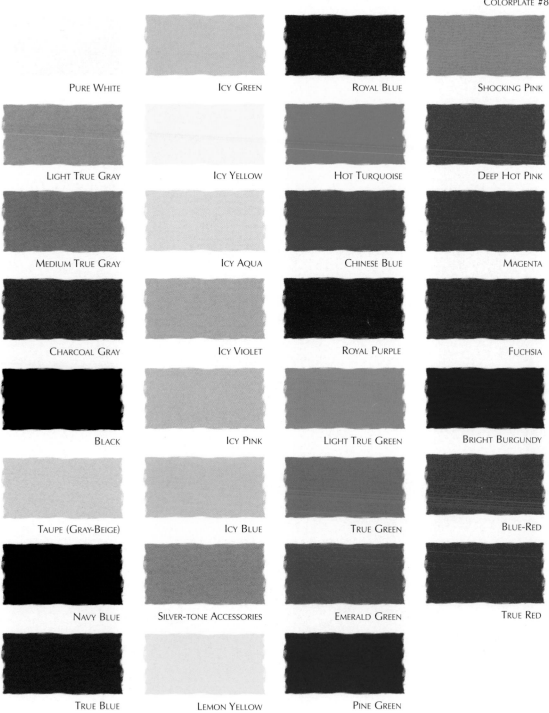

PURE WHITE

ICY GREEN

ROYAL BLUE

SHOCKING PINK

LIGHT TRUE GRAY

ICY YELLOW

HOT TURQUOISE

DEEP HOT PINK

MEDIUM TRUE GRAY

ICY AQUA

CHINESE BLUE

MAGENTA

CHARCOAL GRAY

ICY VIOLET

ROYAL PURPLE

FUCHSIA

BLACK

ICY PINK

LIGHT TRUE GREEN

BRIGHT BURGUNDY

TAUPE (GRAY-BEIGE)

ICY BLUE

TRUE GREEN

BLUE-RED

NAVY BLUE

SILVER-TONE ACCESSORIES

EMERALD GREEN

TRUE RED

TRUE BLUE

LEMON YELLOW

PINE GREEN

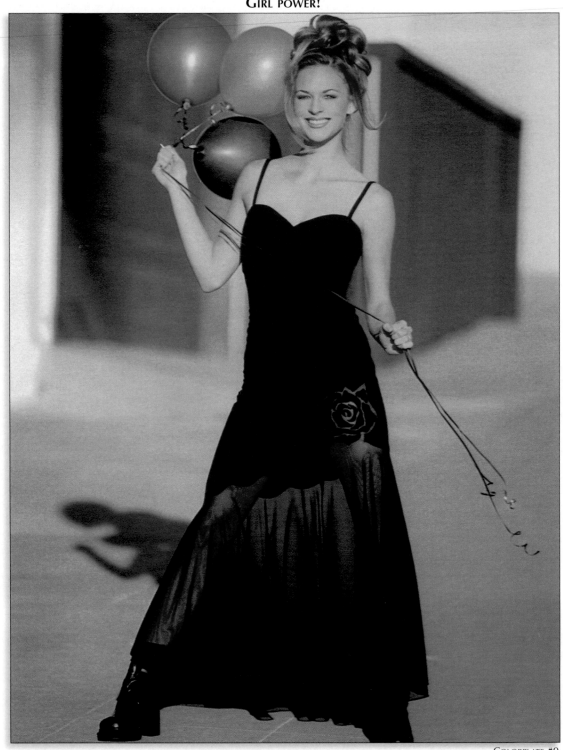

DRESS WITH STYLE—AND PIZZAZZ!

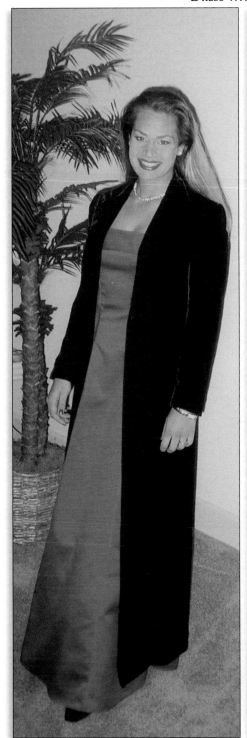

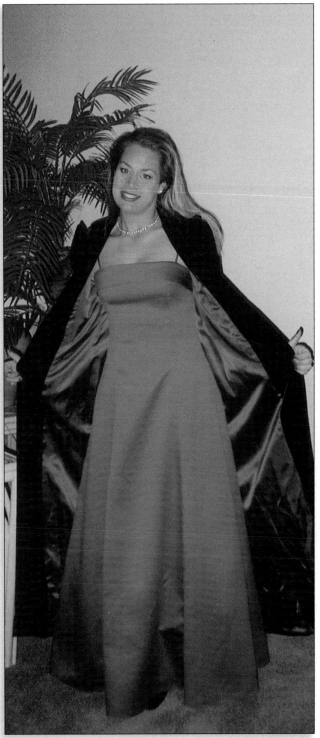

Dress for success . . . and elegance!

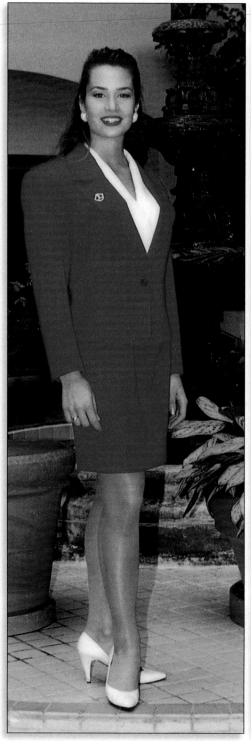

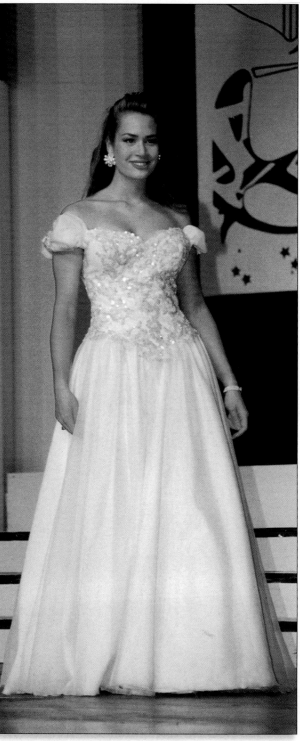

COLORPLATE #12

COLORPLATE #13

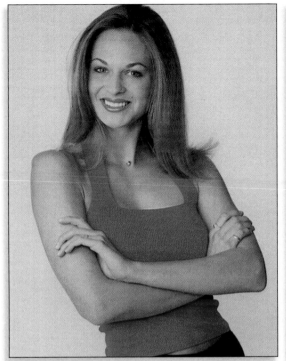

COLORPLATE #14

COLORPLATE #15

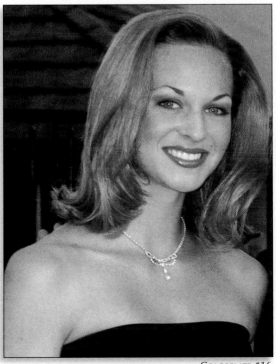

COLORPLATE #16

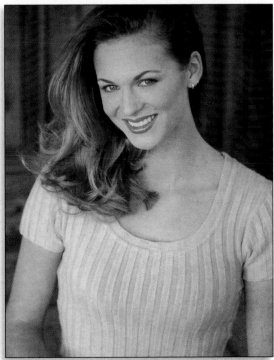

COLORPLATE #17

A Fun Personality Is Always in Style!

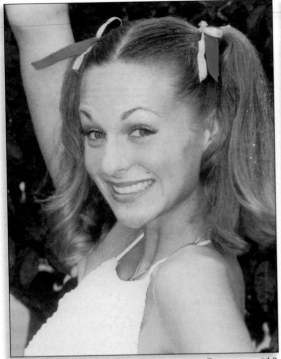

COLORPLATE #18

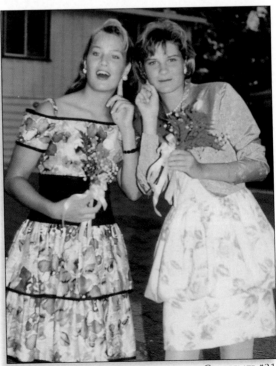

COLORPLATE #19

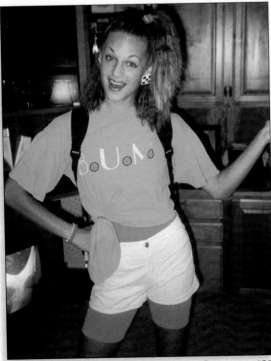

COLORPLATE #20

COLORPLATE #21

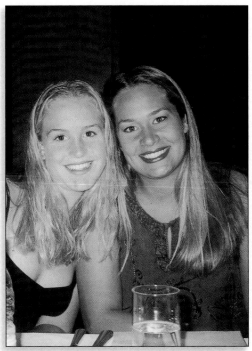

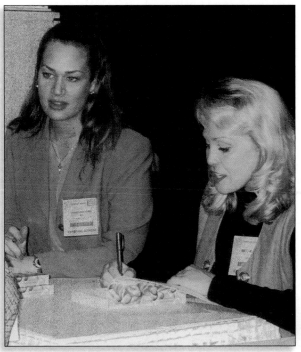

My friend Tina and I in the COLORPLATE #22
Philippines on an Airline Ambassadors
mission delivering humanitarian aid to an orphanage.

Mom and I at an Orlando booksigning COLORPLATE #23
for *Taste Berries for Teens.*

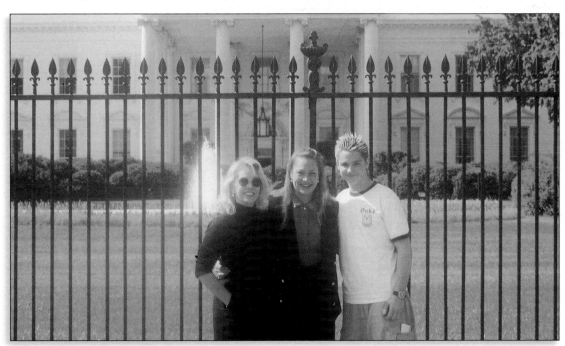

Mom, Josh Levine and I at the White House after an appearance on *Voices of America.* COLORPLATE #24

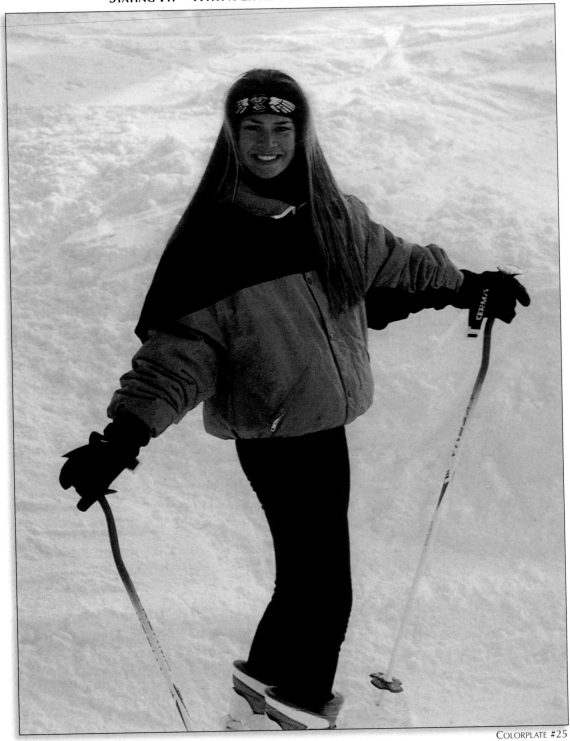

GET INVOLVED!
HELPING OTHERS IS GOOD FOR YOUR HEART AND SOUL

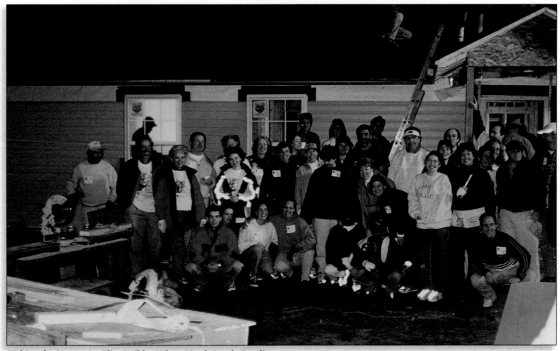

Habitat for Humanity Blitz Build—Hilton Head, South Carolina.

COLORPLATE #26

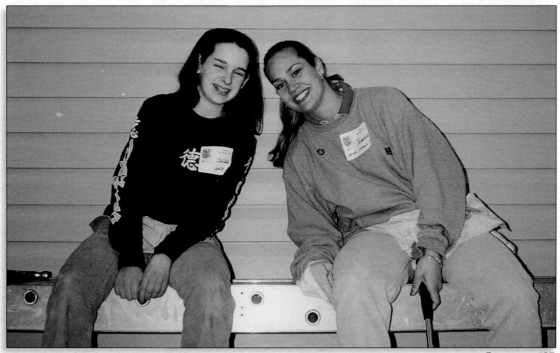

New, and tired, friends at the Habitat Build.

COLORPLATE #27

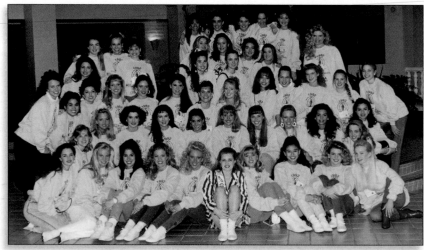

Miss Teen California Contest

COLORPLATE #28

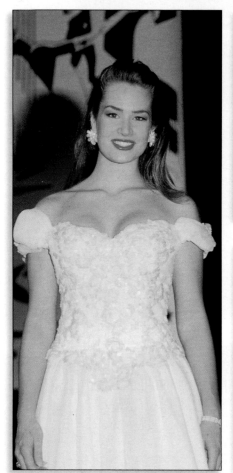

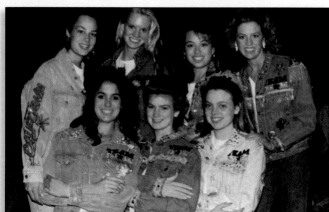

Miss Teen California Semi-Finalists!

COLORPLATE #29

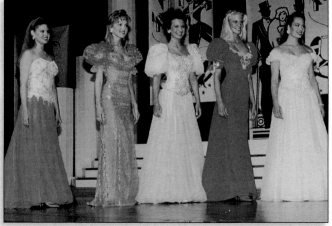

COLORPLATE #30

Miss Teen California Finalists!

COLORPLATE #31

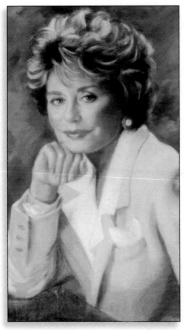
Barbara Walters   Colorplate #32

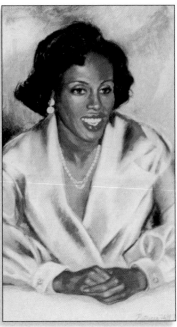
Jackie Joyner-Kersee   Colorplate #33

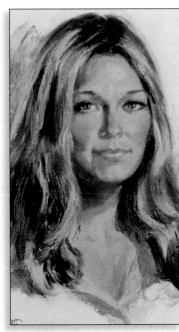
Gloria Steinem   Colorplate #34

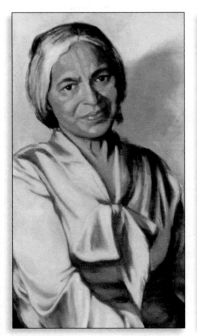
Rosa Parks   Colorplate #35

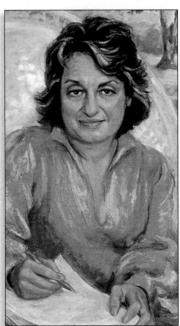
Betty Friedan   Colorplate #36

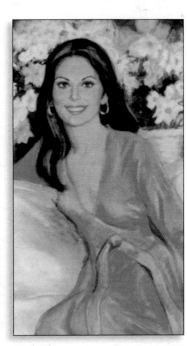
Marlo Thomas   Colorplate #37

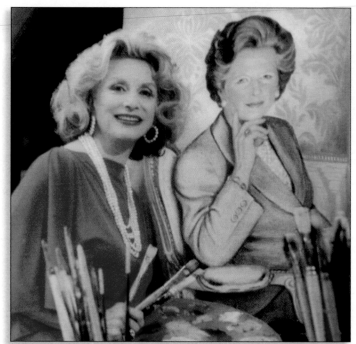

Patricia Hill Burnett with portrait of Margaret Thatcher   COLORPLATE #38

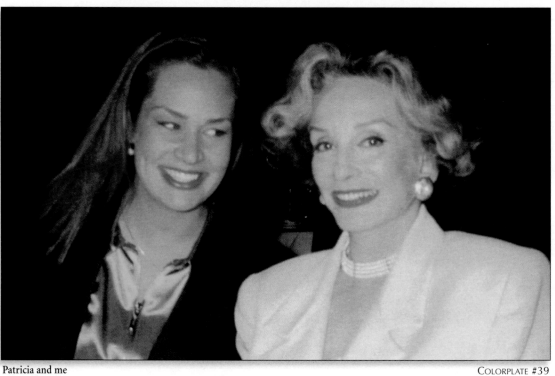

Patricia and me   COLORPLATE #39

SPECIALTY SCARVES BY FRANKIE WELCH OF FRANKIE WELCH DESIGNS

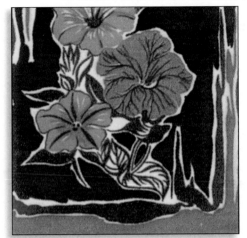

First Lady Betty Ford   COLORPLATE #40

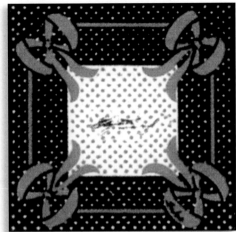

Elizabeth Taylor   COLORPLATE #41

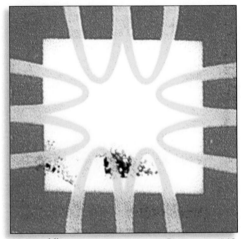

McDonald's   COLORPLATE #42

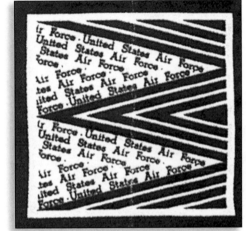

United States Air Force   COLORPLATE #43

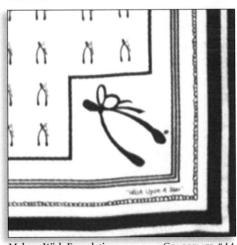

Make-a-Wish Foundation   COLORPLATE #44

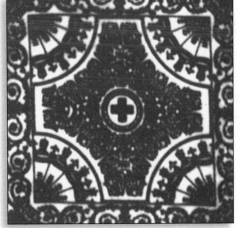

The Red Cross   COLORPLATE #45

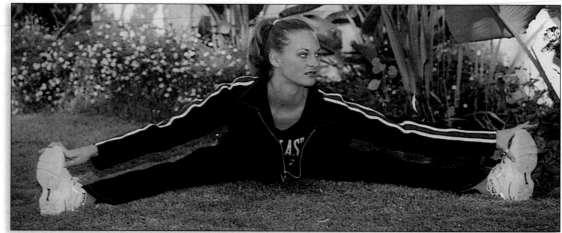

COLORPLATE #46

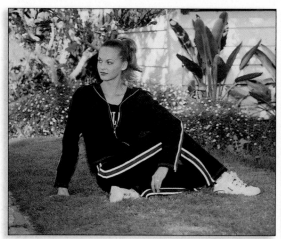

COLORPLATE #47

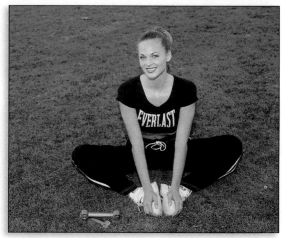

COLORPLATE #48

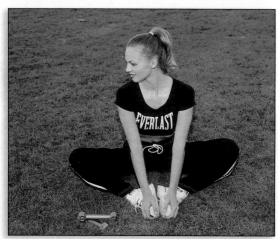

COLORPLATE #49

COLORPLATE #50

Muscles Need Exercise, Too!

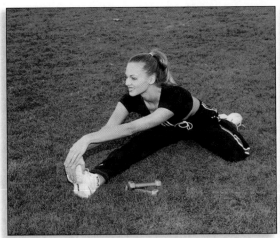

COLORPLATE #51

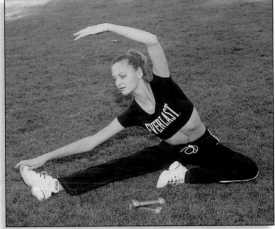

COLORPLATE #52

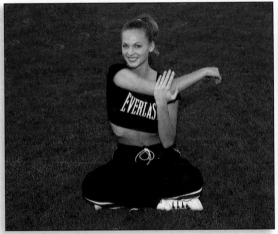

COLORPLATE #53

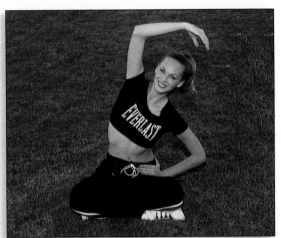

COLORPLATE #54

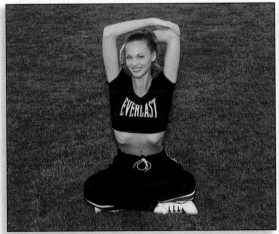

COLORPLATE #55

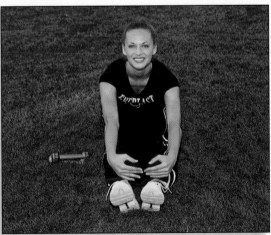

COLORPLATE #56

Computer-Generated Hairstyles of Me by Susan Gilbert of New Looks on Video

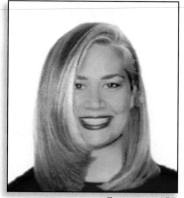

COLORPLATE #57

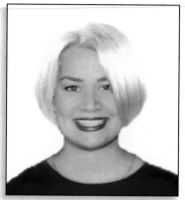

COLORPLATE #58

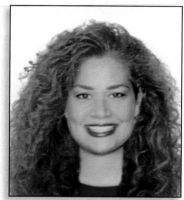

COLORPLATE #59

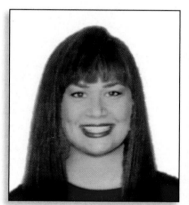

COLORPLATE #60

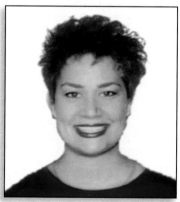

COLORPLATE #61

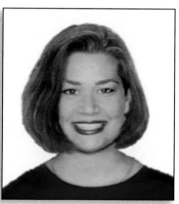

COLORPLATE #62

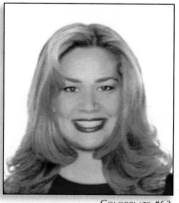

COLORPLATE #63

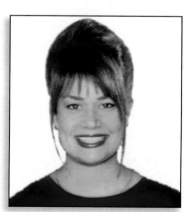

COLORPLATE #64

COMPUTER-GENERATED HAIRSTYLES OF ME BY SUSAN GILBERT OF NEW LOOKS ON VIDEO

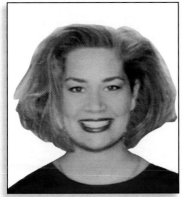

COLORPLATE #65

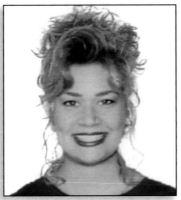

COLORPLATE #66

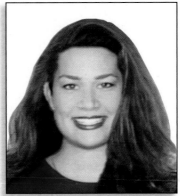

COLORPLATE #67

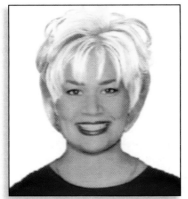

COLORPLATE #68

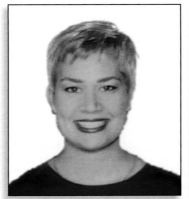

COLORPLATE #69

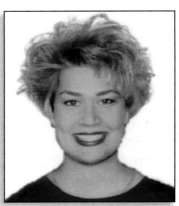

COLORPLATE #70

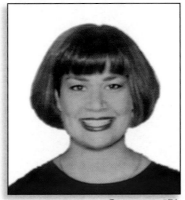

COLORPLATE #71

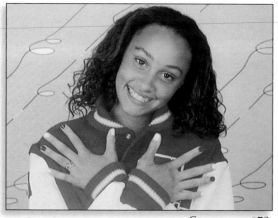

COLORPLATE #72

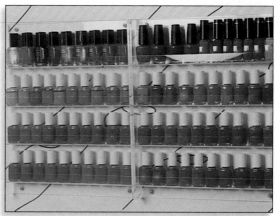

COLORPLATE #73

MAKEUP ARTIST LOIS PEARL AND TEEN CARRIE HAGUE—BEFORE AND AFTER!

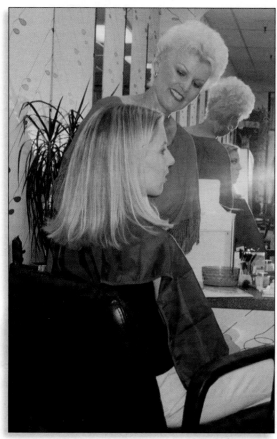

COLORPLATE #74

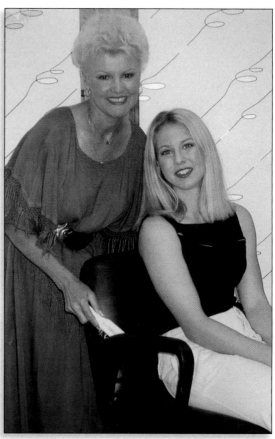

COLORPLATE #75

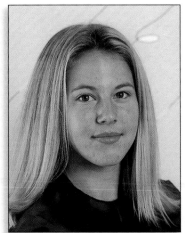

COLORPLATE #76

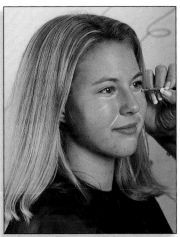

COLORPLATE #77

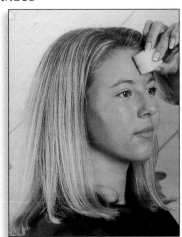

COLORPLATE #78

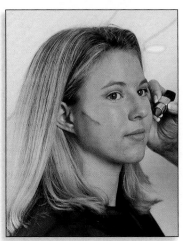

COLORPLATE #79

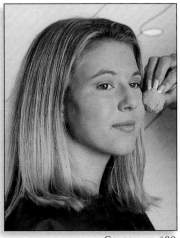

COLORPLATE #80

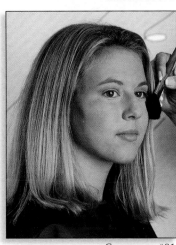

COLORPLATE #81

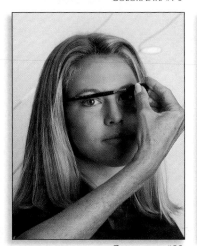

COLORPLATE #82

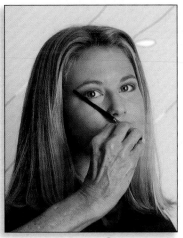

COLORPLATE #83

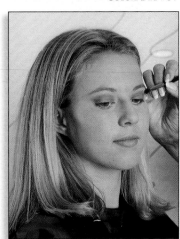

COLORPLATE #84

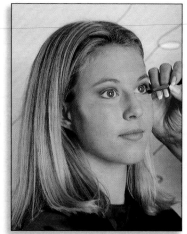

COLORPLATE #85

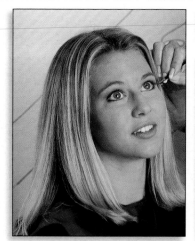

COLORPLATE #86

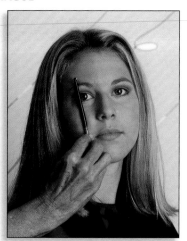

COLORPLATE #87

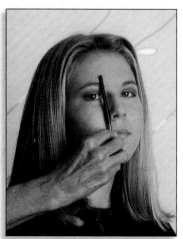

COLORPLATE #88

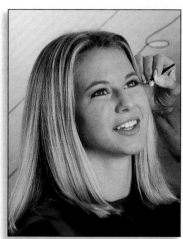

COLORPLATE #89

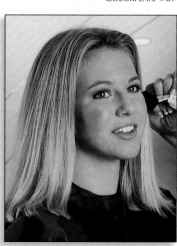

COLORPLATE #90

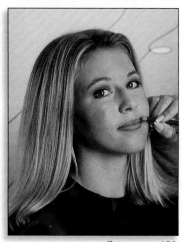

COLORPLATE #91

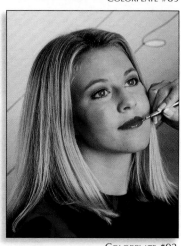

COLORPLATE #92

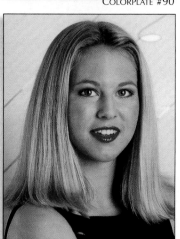

COLORPLATE #93

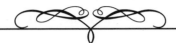

UNIT THREE
Clothes, Colors and Accessories

Think it, talk it, live it, show it.
Whatever you want, whatever you are,
Let the Universe know it!

—MICHAEL DOOLEY

Inventory: Attired and Accented for Beauty— A $1,000 Shopping Spree!

Most girls love to shop. But you know how expensive it is to keep up with all the latest styles and fashions in today's times—and it's no fun to go shopping if you don't have enough money. No problem! Here's $1,000 to spend on any of the following specially priced items. Here's the catch: You only get to choose five items!

❑ A closet full of trendy clothes
❑ A closet full of practical clothes
❑ A closet big enough to hold all my clothes

❏ Clothes in colors that make me look pretty and feel self-confident

❏ My favorite clothes in every fabric imaginable

❏ A closet full of trendy shoes, all styles and colors

❏ A closet full of comfortable shoes

❏ A jewelry box filled with trendy jewelry

❏ A jewelry box filled with practical and special pieces of jewelry

❏ A bottle of all the latest trendy perfumes on the market

❏ Twenty bottles of my one very most favorite perfume

❏ A really cool perfume created just for me

❏ Belts, scarves and purses in every color imaginable

❏ To have just the right touch with accessories

❏ To have a great sense of style

❏ To have a look all my own, one that others always remark on, saying how cool I look

❏ To be one of those girls who looks great in everything she wears

❏ To be as clothes savvy as some of the girls I know

❏ A fashion makeover by the world's very top fashion designer

❏ A shopping spree like this, every month

Did you have a lot of fun on this spending spree? Who wouldn't, right? But let's take your spending spree a little further. Look back over the five items you selected. With number one being your first choice, put them in their order of importance to you. Pretty tough to do, right? That's because our needs are dependent upon our lifestyles. Look again at the priorities you listed. They can tell you a lot about your clothing and the accessories you may need, whether you think so or not. This unit will show you how to shop wisely and is sure to get you on the "most impressive" list at your school!

12

What Your Appearance Tells Others About You

There is no beauty that hath not some
strangeness in its proportion.

—FRANCIS BACON

Do You Judge a Book by Its Cover?

"Don't judge a book by its cover" is an honorable virtue most of us aspire to, but, oftentimes we still end up forming an impression based upon how someone looks. I remember the first time I met Brad, whom you met in chapter 1. He was smartly dressed in clean, pressed khaki pants, a mod white-and-blue shirt, fashionable woven leather sandals, with trendy sunglasses smartly perched atop his well-groomed head of hair. Bright eyes, a friendly smile and gleaming teeth completed the look.

One glance and I decided that here was a contemporary guy, one who knew what looked good on him and cared enough about himself to take the time to look good. His appearance made me think:

"This guy's in tune with his appearance. He's current."

"This guy's immaculately groomed. I'll bet he keeps his car clean and his apartment tidy."

"This guy's outgoing. He's probably got a lot of nice friends."

"This guy's into dental hygiene. I'll bet he's a good kisser!"

Though I didn't know Brad at the time, the style and manner in which he was dressed, along with his friendly demeanor, gave me all those impressions. Now, after having dated him for some seven months, I've discovered that what his appearance "told me" was true!

Chinos Chatter, Tommy Tattles: Clothes Talk

Does someone's appearance influence how you think about him or her? I have to admit—that was the case for me with Brad. A person's appearance can't tell you "who" that person is, nor should it ever be a basis for judging a person's character, but it makes an impression nonetheless.

If, as they say, a picture is worth a thousand words, then my school was a colossal picture-book dictionary. Cheryl *always* dressed provocatively. She wore her skirts very short, and tank tops, T-shirts and blouses that were much too tight and revealing. To this she added large platform shoes and sometimes high heels. My friends thought the way she dressed wasn't in very good taste for school, as well as thinking it would be uncomfortable having to spend an entire day in those things. Her appearance made us feel uncomfortable—in more ways than one. Because of the way she dressed, the "nice" girls—while polite to her—kept their distance, never including her in any of their activities in school, nor inviting her to join them when they wanted to just hang out after school or on the weekends.

If Cheryl was clueless about the fact that the way she dressed made some of us girls hesitate to be her friends, she was even more oblivious to the fact that while most all the boys in our school flirted with her, none of the boys with a "good reputation" ever asked her out. (They didn't want to be seen with her because if they were, none of the "nice" girls would go out with them.) Nor could she ever figure out why the only boys who did ask her out were those who were rumored to "want only one thing."

Megan had a "reputation" for the way she dressed, too. Megan was an artsy and whimsical girl with an outgoing personality who dressed mostly in bold prints and vibrant colors. Everyone knew that one day Megan would be somebody *special* in the art world. She looked the part. One of her outfits that was a favorite of mine was an ankle-length flowing skirt with contrasting geometric shapes in various shades of blue, purple and rose, worn with a softly shaped, very long ivory sweater. To this she added an eye-catching choker of painted wooden blocks with a matching oversized bracelet. I don't know where she shopped, but Megan had a knack for finding the most unusual shoes and artsy-craftsy jewelry. It was easy to tell from her appearance that Megan was creative and artistic—she used herself as a canvas, creating a picture that showcased her talent more than any brochure or business card could.

Sara was a shy and demure girl, her clothes reflecting a gentle and soft-spoken personality. In her yearbook she listed her ambition as wanting to teach elementary school. I thought she would probably make a good teacher for small children, especially with her reverent way of being such an attentive listener—an eye for detail that also showed up in the way she dressed. She preferred soft fabrics and small floral prints and wore mostly one-piece dresses and blouses and slacks—never jeans. Sara loved soft pastels, a real contrast to Marriah, an outgoing and flamboyant girl—just like her wardrobe.

Marriah loved bright colors and nappy fabrics. Always dramatic, Marriah wore interesting clothes and bold jewelry that matched her confidence. She told everyone she wanted "her own company." None of us doubted that one day she would have a business of her own, even if no one (including Marriah) knew just what the nature of her company might be!

Comfort was my thing. In my school, team players wore a jersey on the day of a game. Basically this was the school's display of spirit and an alert to other students that today a certain team was playing and they should head for the bleachers and support their friends rather than head off to McDonald's or the mall. I played three sports each year, so I was often in a uniform. When I wasn't, I still dressed in casual clothes because when I went to practice, which was usually every day after school, I knew that the clothes I wore to school that day were going to end up at the bottom of my sports bag, and I probably would not unpack them until much later that evening—or, quite possibly, until a day or two later! So, I picked my clothes for comfort, wear and easy wash.

I'm quite sure no one ever thought of me as glamorous (well, maybe Ben!) but, rather, just your average "girl next door nice friend." Or at least I think that's what they thought. I was chosen "Most Inspirational Player" for three years in a row, even when I sometimes felt that another student deserved it as much, and even when I didn't think I'd get chosen since I had won the award the year before. Thinking back, I think I was seen as an athlete partly because of the casual and sporty way I dressed.

No doubt about it, the clothes we wear—and the way we wear them— create an impression, one that others can readily see.

What Do _Your_ Clothes Say About You?

What does your appearance say about you? Are you shy or outspoken? Gregarious or laid-back? Are you sporty, artsy, an intellectual? Think about this for a moment and then in the spaces provided below, jot down several words you think best describe what your appearance reveals about you.

My appearance tells others that I am a person who _____

_____.

Now ask a couple of good friends to describe what they think your appearance says about you. You might also ask your mom or dad. The goal is to see what others think and to see how their views compare to yours.

Now comes another very important question: What do you *want* your appearance to tell others about you? Think about this for a moment, and then see if you can express it in writing. Go ahead and try this now.

I'd like my appearance to tell others that I am a person who _____

_____.

Study your words for a minute and reflect upon them. Is your appearance giving off the message you would like it to?

Sending Your Message with "Style"

Also evident in your appearance is your sense of style. Style is more than dressing in the latest fad or fashion or wearing expensive fabrics or intricately tailored designs. Style is about a sense of self and becomes a classic way you have of presenting yourself to the world.

The late Audrey Hepburn, a style legend, reigned as a movie star of the 1950s and 1960s. In addition to being an accomplished actress, one of Ms. Hepburn's greatest starring roles is that of the public's ideal of someone with a supreme sense of style. As a result, her name is practically synonymous with glamour. She is considered one of the great beauties of all time. Yet she wasn't beautiful in the classic way we think of beauty. It's just that she had such a way about her, a ladylike and soft-spoken elegance. And, she possessed a

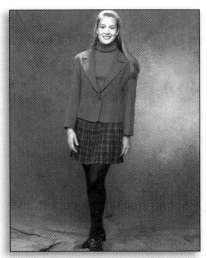

Style projects a sense of self.

sense of fashion that was elegance personified. Perhaps one day her name will be replaced by recording artist Celine Dion, actress and singer Brandy, fashion model Kim Alexis or someone else who displays such a wonderful sense of class and style.

Style, you see, is not about *being* beautiful as much as projecting a beautiful sense of self. [See colorplates 10–17.]

Dara Montgomery— Our Very Own Audrey Hepburn

Dara Montgomery was my school's Audrey Hepburn. Dara could pull together a fabulous outfit like no one else I knew. She just seemed to have a natural talent for choosing what went with what. Be it the day of school pictures or the day our school attended a lecture at a local museum, a sporting event or the prom, Dara showed up smartly dressed for the occasion, and she always wore an outfit that complemented the activity at hand.

It wasn't just Dara's knowing what to wear and when to wear it that made her stand out and seem so much more "with it" than the rest of us. She didn't spend a lot of money on her clothes, nor did she necessarily have a lot of clothes. Dara had a keen fashion sense about what looked good on her and why. She had a knack for combining certain pieces with others in a way that really worked, and an eye for mixing and matching certain colors that complemented her coloring and features.

I distinctly recall watching Dara walk up to the front of the class one day to hand in a paper, looking as though she could have been a fashion consultant in a nice department store. She was wearing a deep sea-green sweater with a pleated plaid skirt that swayed loosely as she moved. Draped around her shoulders was a rather large, bold rust-colored scarf. Knotted in a really unique way, it hung down to her waist. As always, she smelled of gardenias, a fragrance as clean and simple as the understated silver jewelry she wore. Just a hint of rust eye-shadow and a subdued shade of lip gloss finished off "her look," one that made Dara appear poised, centered and complete—as usual. Dara's look of being "polished, poised, centered and complete," was her style, always evident in whatever she was wearing at any given time. We understood that Dara knew something about clothes the rest of us didn't.

We can all learn Dara's secrets of style.

The Secret to Creating a Style of Your Own

Looking through fashion magazines is one good way to develop an awareness of style. Observing others around you is an even better method, since the people we see in our everyday lives are more likely to be those with whom we wish to fit in. Tune in to what others are wearing and how a certain style or color makes them look. See if you can determine what it is about another's appearance that you like—or don't like—and why. Ask yourself:

- Does the person's appearance project an overall look that is attractive? If so, give your reasons. For example, you might think, "She looks neat and well-groomed"; "she looks 'together'"; "she looks comfortable."
- Does the particular style the person is wearing look good on her? Again, give your reasons. For example, "That skirt length flatters her height."

- Does the color of the outfit flatter her? If so, why? If not, what color do you think would? For example, "That deep purple suit is a great color for her, much better than a lighter lavender, which would seem washed out next to her dark hair, eyes and complexion." Or, "The pastel sweater looks very nice with her pale complexion and sandy-blonde hair."
- Do the accessories she is wearing look good with her outfit, do they complement the garments she is wearing? If so, why? If not, what do you think would look better? For example, "I think a black patent belt would look better than the black leather belt she is wearing." Again, offer an explanation for your reason, for example, "Since she is wearing black patent shoes, a matching belt would be more pleasing to the eye and tie her outfit together."

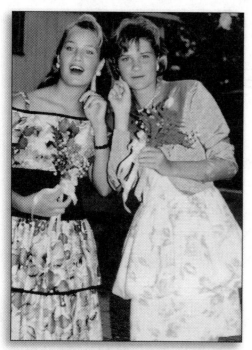

An awareness of how certain styles, colors and accessories complement the appearances of others can sharpen your own fashion sense. That's why when you're studying what does or doesn't look good on others, it's important to do more than say, "Wow, she looks great," or, "That really looks awful on her." Try to figure out why something either does or doesn't work. This is information you can use to determine how certain styles, fabrics and colors might look on you.

Choosing styles that work well with your body shape, and wearing colors that are most flattering to your hair and skin tone, not only show you have a fashion sense about you, but they are steps in the right direction toward helping you look your very best.

The next few chapters will show you how. [Also see colorplates 28–31.]

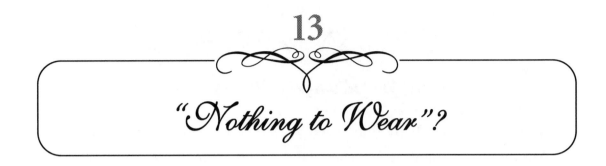

"Nothing to Wear"?

Beauty is all very well at first sight.
But who ever looks at it when it has been
in the house for three days?

—SAPPHO

Singing the Nothing-to-Wear Blues

How many times each weekday do you need to look your *best?* There's the group photo for band on Wednesday, a job interview at a store in the mall Thursday after school, and you're hoping a special guy will take notice when you casually ask whether or not he's got a date for the upcoming dance. Almost every day, you have a reason to look *just right*. And almost as often, you rummage through your closet searching for the perfect outfit to wear, but nothing feels right. You try on dress after pants after skirt, posing in front of the mirror and sighing in despair. "I have nothing to wear!" you moan—only to be reminded by your mother, "You have a closet full of clothes!"

You know she's right. So how is it you can't find anything that looks or feels right?

So, Why Don't You Have Anything to Wear?

If you identify with the nothing-to-wear blues, you aren't alone. From Maine to Spain, from the islands to the heartland, teens tell me they have nothing to wear! Do you have "nothing to wear" because: You look like a fire engine in the red sweater you bought last month; the new style of pants that made your best friend look really cool makes you look positively awful; you loaned out your favorite skirt and your friend has not returned it; the pale yellow blouse you thought you'd love doesn't go with anything in your closet; your brown belt is the wrong shade to wear with your slacks; you don't have a single pair of shoes that looks good with your new dress? If so, of course you have nothing to wear!

If you're like the rest of us, you cry that you have "nothing to wear!" when, in reality, you:

✓ Forget about some of the things you have.

✓ Don't like the way certain things fit you.

✓ Are tired of wearing that one "standby" outfit—the one that is so comfortable and looks good for all occasions that you reach for it time and time again.

✓ Forget to launder garments when needed so an item is not clean on the day you want to wear it.

✓ Don't like the color of a certain item.

✓ Don't want to wear the garments that are now out of style.

✓ Can't keep track of what you've loaned out and to whom.

✓ Just want an excuse to buy something more.

Your Closet:
Home for the Perfect Wardrobe

A good way to get a handle on the nothing-to-wear blues is to take inventory. The goal is to think about all the clothes, belts and shoes you already own—your wardrobe. Identify *all* the clothes and shoes in your closet and your dresser drawers, your clothes hamper, in the trunk of your (or your parents') car, the laundry room, as well as those that may be hanging in your best friend's closet. Don't forget the loose shoe or article or two of clothing that may have tried to run away and are now hiding under your bed. And don't forget those items you've been meaning to retrieve from the "Lost and Found" bin at school, as well as any other place you could have left certain items. By assessing your wardrobe, you will know what you own but don't wear—and why—and can better determine what you need in order to wear other pieces.

At the end of this chapter you will find a Clothing Inventory worksheet. The inventory is designed to help you itemize all the clothing, belts, shoes and accessories you have. This inventory will help you get a very clear picture of your wardrobe so you'll get a better idea why you don't like or don't wear certain pieces—all of which can be a big reason you "don't have anything to wear."

The inventory can be helpful because it:

• Is a good visual—a way to see all the items you have.

• Helps clarify why you may not be wearing certain pieces but would *if only* (you had the right pair of pants, the right kind of shoes, a white T-shirt, and so on).

• Helps you remember items that you've forgotten all about having, and to get new ideas for coordinating different articles of clothing.

• Helps determine what items to give away or "trade" with a friend who likes the garment.

- Helps you identify what you need so that you can ask for a certain item as a birthday gift, or know what to look for the next time you go shopping.

Sasha Linn's Inventory

The inventory of Sasha Linn, a teen from Shreveport, Louisiana, appears on the following pages. Glance through it so that you will have an idea how yours will look after you've completed it. (Even if you go to a school or have a job that requires a uniform or dress code, complete the inventory.)

As you are looking over Sasha's inventory, notice the four columns: item, fabric, color and comments. Also notice the general headings under *items:* pants, skirts, dresses, blouses, sweaters, jackets, Ts, jumpers, shoes, belts and accessories. Itemizing your things according to *kind* is a good way to see exactly what you have and can pinpoint reasons why you may or may not be wearing certain things. For example, let's say you're getting ready for school and decide you'll wear that great new top you bought over the weekend. So you pull on the new top and then search for a pair of slacks to wear with it—but feel nothing looks quite right. "I have no pants!" you declare. But in fact, you have ten pairs of slacks and jeans! You just don't have a pair that would look really great with your new top! If you knew exactly what you owned prior to shopping, you would have known that you should have also shopped for a pair of slacks or skirt to wear with your new top—or purchased some other top instead, one that would go with a pair of slacks (or skirt) you already owned. I'll explain the fabric, color and comments columns later in this chapter. Right now, look over Sasha's inventory to get a feel for how it works.

Sasha's Clothing Inventory

Item	Fabric	Color	Comments
PANTS			
Capri	Cotton/spandex	Beige	Very comfortable
Overalls	Cotton	Blue	Very comfortable
Slacks	Don't know	Black	Starting to show wear
Blue jeans	Denim	Black	Too small, tight
Blue jeans	Denim	Light blue	Look great with Ts
Blue jeans	Denim	Faded blue	Live in these; great fit
Pants (casual)	Twill	Blue	Matching jacket
Khaki pants	Khaki	Beige	Comfortable; look great
Blue jeans	Denim	Faded blue	Holes in knees, butt area Can wear only sometimes
Blue jeans	Denim	Red	Don't like
Blue jeans	Denim	Dark blue	Don't like style
SKIRTS			
Straight flowered	Cotton	Multi	Casual—looks good with T-shirts
Ankle length	Cotton	Multi br/gold	Western look; have to be really in the mood to wear
Short skirt	Don't know	Navy	Love it! My dance skirt
Short skirt	Denim	Flowered	Looks great with Ts
Full skirt	Linen	Blue	Ruined in the wash!

Item	Fabric	Color	Comments
SKIRTS (continued)			
Mini	Don't know	Black	Mom won't let me wear any longer; still love it
Mini	Denim	Faded blue	Too small, outgrown
DRESSES			
Casual long	Polyester	Flowers	Wear to church a lot
Knee length, Decorative buttons	Cotton knit	Deep Blue	A great dress-up look; my "first date" dress
Formal two-piece	Wool	Hunter Green	Works with dressy blouse, too
Sundress	Cotton	Multi	Can wear in summer only
BLOUSES			
Long sleeves	Cotton	White	I live in this
Striped long-sleeve shirt	Cotton	Black/White	Looks great with jeans
Short sleeves	Cotton	Yellow	Should give away
Long sleeves	Cotton	White	Showing wear
SWEATERS			
Long sleeves	Knit	Ivory	Goes with almost everything
	Present from Aunt Sue	Purple	Makes me look like a big grape
	Knit	Tan	Great with long skirt
	Acrylic	Stripes	Don't like
Cropped cardigan	Don't know	Black	Really like

Item	Fabric	Color	Comments
JACKETS			
	Twill	Blue	Matching pants
School logo	Leather	Black	Couldn't live without it!
	Denim	Blue	Must get back from Erin
	Denim	Black	Where is this?
	Denim	White	Doesn't go with anything!
Ts			
	Cotton	White	Own four! Live in these!
	Cotton	Black	Live in this!
	Cotton	White	Very washed out
Drake University logo	Cotton	Yellow	New! Love it! Got it while attending Drake Relays
School logo	Cotton	Navy	Wear to school games
JUMPERS			
Knee length	Don't know	Beige	Boring; never did like
Ankle length	Nylon	Dark Brown	Boring, but wear a lot
Mini	Denim	Faded Blue	Wear on library days
V-neck	Linen	Sand	Always looks wrinkled
SHOES			
Air Jordans	Canvas	White	Wear them three times a week!
NineWest	Leather	Brown	Love 'em
Tennis	Canvas	White	Love 'em
Nike Swoops	Canvas	White/Black	Great to wear!

Item	Fabric	Color	Comments
SHOES *(continued)*			
Loafers	Leather	Brown	Wear a lot
Casual slip-ons	Upper is cloth	Beige	Wear with skirts
Heels	Leather	Black	Wear for dress-up
Loafers	Leather	Navy	Not very comfortable
Heels	Leather, I think	Floral	Don't go with anything
Heels	Cloth	Pink	From my sister's wedding. Dye black for prom dress?
BELTS			
	Western	Black	Wear it all the time
	Leather stitch	Black	Wear a lot
	Cloth	Black	Worn out, holes stretched
	Leather	Black	Too small
	Plastic	White	Ugly; never wear
	Patent Leather	Black	Wear a lot
	Woven Leather	Navy	Fallen apart
	Leather	Red	Too small
	Leather	White	Too short for low-waisted pants and skirts
ACCESSORIES/RINGS			
Class ring		Gold	Never take off
Assorted (10)			Junky, almost never wear

Item	Fabric	Color	Comments
NECKLACES			
Fake pearls			Mostly wear to church (also wore to prom)
Assorted (5)			I really don't like to wear necklaces
Lots of "junk"			Not even my little sister wants these! Old, tarnished, tangled
EARRINGS			
Fake pearls			Matches necklace
Gold loops (4 pr)			Live in these
Others (8 pr)			Out of style; tarnished
BRACELETS			
Gold			Wear on dates sometimes
Assortment (8)			I don't like to wear bracelets

How to Inventory Your Wardrobe

Okay, so that's the idea. As you can see from looking over Sasha's inventory, it's a pretty straightforward task. Now it's your turn.

You'll find your copy of the Clothing Inventory at the end of this chapter. Since you'll be needing it as you go through the next several chapters, complete it as soon as you can. It's probably going to take you a good hour or so, so you may want to schedule doing it at a time when you can put on your favorite CD and plow in. It would also be a fun activity to do with your very best friend.

Here's a suggestion: You may want to make a copy of this worksheet before you complete it so that you'll have an extra copy to use when you'd like to take stock of your things again. You may even want to give a copy of it to a friend, so she can inventory her things, as well. (You can also create your own inventory just by using lined notebook paper.)

Here are the steps:

Step 1: Under the column *Pants,* list your favorite pair.

Step 2: The next column is *Fabric.* Jot down the material or fabric.

Step 3: The next column is *Color.* Write down the color of this pair of pants.

Step 4: The next column is *Comments.* Here add a comment as to what you like or dislike about the item of clothing, such as "love it!" or "makes me look and feel great!" or "needs hemming," or "loaned to a friend," or "need to get back," and so on. Be as thorough as you can.

Step 5: Now list your next-favorite pair of pants, or the one you wear the most, and then list the fabric, color and comment. Do this for each pair of pants you have, beginning with the ones you wear and like the most, working your way down to listing those you wear the least—or not at all.

Step 6: Do this for each and every item in your closet.

Step 7: Inventory your shoes, belts, jewelry and accessories, including handbags if you own more than a couple.

Any Surprises?

Once the inventory is completed, review it carefully. Are you surprised by the length of your itemized list? Do you have a lot of clothes, or not as many as you thought? Do you notice anything telling? For example, do you have several favorite garments, such as short skirts, that you don't presently wear *because* you don't have the right kinds of shoes to wear with them? Or, now that your best white blouse has a big mustard stain on it, do your favorite skirts hang week after week, month after month, without being worn? Or, are there three or more items on the list you noted as "out of style"?

In the next few chapters I'll address some of the most common "closet quandaries," such as, "I don't like the way it looks on me," and "The color is all wrong!" and help you discover why that is, and what you can do to dress with style, class and pizzazz!

Don't forget to keep your Clothing Inventory handy! You'll need it as you read throughout the rest of this unit.

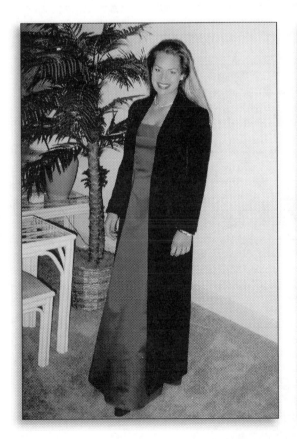
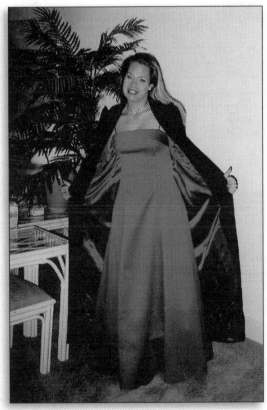

Your Personal Clothing Inventory

Name: _____ Date: _____

Item	Fabric	Color	Comments

What Looks Best on _Your_ Body?

_**T**he perception of beauty
is a moral test._

—HENRY DAVID THOREAU

Do Your Clothes Look Good on You?

In reviewing the comments column of your Clothing Inventory, did you find that one of the reasons you don't wear a certain item or favorite outfit is because "I don't like the way it looks on me"? For teens, that's the number-one complaint as to why an article of clothing shows up at the bottom of their list.

If a certain article of clothing doesn't look quite right on you, why is that? Is it because you have outgrown it, or that you don't like the color? Is it because it reminds you of a time when you spent a lot of time with a certain friend— who is no longer your friend? Or is it that you don't have the right body for the outfit—or, rather, that the outfit simply isn't designed for _your_ body?

Maybe it doesn't look quite right on you because it's _not_ really right for you.

Every girl can wear skirts, pants and dresses. We just can't all wear the _same_ skirts, pants and dresses. How we look in something is often determined by our shape, and more precisely, our _body line_.

Do You Have a "Perfect" Body?

Girls are often overly critical about their shape. It's one of the most common complaints I hear from teens. When I was in a Miss Teen California Pageant—surrounded by healthy, fit and beautiful girls—I heard it then, too. Contestant after contestant remarked to each other, "I wish I had your figure!" or "I wish I were as tall as you!" or "I wish I were as beautiful as you!" or "You're so perfect!" And of course, I caught myself saying the same things to them.

"Perfect body" stereotypes feed off our insecurities, and only serve to make us unhappy with our own natural beauty. Besides, our ideal of "perfect" constantly changes. The "it girl" of the 1950s was Marilyn Monroe, petite and voluptuous. In today's time, Ms. Monroe would probably be considered slightly overweight. In the 1960s a model called Twiggy set the standard, and every girl longed to be tall and thin as a reed. In today's time, we would probably consider Twiggy to have a weight problem, too—anorexia! The mid- to late-1980s brought us Madonna—five feet, five inches, fit, toned, savvy and sassy—while the early 1990s ushered in Cindy Crawford, followed by the minimalist look with bone-thin models like Kate Moss. This was followed by the wholesome and healthy looks of a bevy of beauties like Drew Barrymore and the Spice Girls who showed us that a rounded tummy can be as healthy—and flattering—as a taut one. There's always a new "it girl," each one escorting a new ideal of "perfect."

How to Be the New "It Girl"

Even if your school's "it girl" is very different from you, instead of trying to become her, work with what you have. By studying your features and body lines, you can learn how to dress in a way that complements or plays up your best features, while downplaying or detracting attention from those things you don't like as much. Again, a reminder: In the teen years, your body is still growing and changing. Enjoy the styles you can wear now. And be ready to leave them behind when it's time to move on.

Understanding your "body line" is a first step in selecting clothing that is most flattering to *you*.

Your "Body Line"— And What It Means

A remark such as "I'm tall" or "I'm short" may be a good way of describing your height, but it's only one part of the picture when it comes to describing your body shape. If you were to add "I'm small-boned" or "I'm large-boned," that would be another piece, but it still isn't enough. Nor is mentioning how much you weigh. A more important consideration is the shape of your body. The question, "Are you more *straight* or *rounded?*" offers more useful information in determining what styles look best on you.

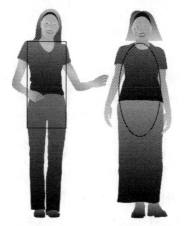

Straight Body Shape　　**Curved Body Shape**

In chapter 9, "What You Should Know About Losing Weight," you met two girls. Each weighs 112 pounds, but Karen is seven inches taller than Rianna. Do you think they both look good in the same styles? Probably not.

If we compare Rianna's body line with the drawing on the previous page, she would fall into the "round" category. Rianna has a rounded shape, whereas Karen has straight bones—her shape is more like the shape of a boy. Neither girl can change her bone structure, but they can dress in those styles that help them achieve the look each of them wants.

Which of the two body types do you think best describes you? Go ahead, see if you know. My body line is:

❏ More straight than curvy

❏ More curvy than straight

How to Determine the True Shape of Your Body

We often think we know the shape of our bodies. But when you try this next exercise, you'll see how different even our own perceptions of our bodies can be from what we think they are.

A good way to determine your shape or "body line," as professional tailors call it, is to trace the outline of your body. The result is a visual that can reveal a great deal of information, one you can use in thinking about the styles that look best on your frame. Tape a large sheet of paper to a wall—the kind that's used to cover tables—and then ask your mom or a good friend to use a marker pen to trace around your body. Trace from head to toes. Then stand back and look at the outline of the figure you see.

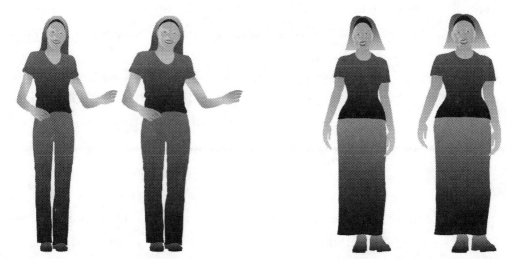

If you gain or lose twenty-five or even fifty pounds, your basic body line will not change. If your body line is straight, it will remain straight. If your body line is curved, it will remain curved. Selecting clothing with the same or similar shape as your body line is the first step in becoming well dressed.

You may be surprised at what you find. When my friend Jessica did this, she was surprised to discover an outline that revealed a "straight body" without much of a waistline or hips. "I honestly thought of myself differently than what the picture revealed," Jessica remarked. "I was always trying to gain weight so that I could have hips. But I can see from the outline that I do have hips, it's just that I have virtually no waistline. My body is a perfect balance of 'straight.' I've decided to declare a truce with my body and rid myself of the negative feeling of not liking my shape. I'm better off learning how to choose clothes that flatter my bone structure and body lines. By wearing the styles that flatter me, I can still achieve the look I want."

Jessica has discovered the key to looking really good in clothes: Your body line is an important consideration in selecting clothes that look good on your body type.

Dress to Complement the Perfect Body—Yours!

Regardless of your shape, whether you have straight lines and wish you had a curved shape or have a curved shape and wish you had straight lines, by learning how to select clothes that complement your shape, you can look sharp and stylish.

It's not possible to go into all the variations on how to select the clothes that are ideal for your body type in this chapter. My intent is help you understand the principle behind dressing with your body lines in mind. For example, fashion experts have determined that if your body lines are more straight than curvy, then:

- Straight styles in plain colors or linear prints (stripes and plaids) will look best on you.
- Accessories and jewelry in rectangular or geometric shapes are made for you.
- If you are large-boned or on the heavy side, larger patterns and accessories work well on you. You can compensate with vertical lines.

On the other hand, if your body lines are more curvy than straight, then:

- A jacket with a fitted waist brings out the beauty of your natural shapeliness.
- Plain colors and prints are more flattering to you than stripes or plaids.
- Accessories in rounded earrings and necklace shapes suit you best.

If you are small-boned and petite, then:

- You can wear small prints or thin stripes well.
- You look better in small earrings and lockets on thin chains.
- Wide stripes or huge prints and big earrings that are flattering to a larger person will completely overpower you.

Some clothing shapes, such as those with a softened line that are neither too straight nor too curved, work well for both curved and straight body types. Try it and you will see that you and your mirror agree.

Again, this is only the tip of the information available to help you dress your very best. The suggested reading section in the back of this book provides additional sources of information to help you learn more. Additionally, most major department stores employ fashion consultants and personal shoppers. This is a good source of advice, as well. And don't forget your home economics and life skills courses at school. Information pertinent to understanding the principles of style was offered in my school. Check to see if it is offered at yours.

How to Play Up Your Best Features —And Minimize Your Flaws

The good news is that you can almost always maximize the effect of your best features and minimize the ones you don't like. Below are just a few of the ways to play up your best features and camouflage others—to make your "flaws" work to your advantage.

Neck

Problem: My neck is too long.
Solution: Wear turtlenecks, scarves or chokers to shorten its appearance.
Problem: My neck is too short.
Solution: A scoop, V-neckline or an open collar will make it appear longer. Vertical features, such as long necklaces, scarves and bows tied low, or ruffles down the front of your blouse, will also give the image of a longer neck.

Shoulders

Problem: My shoulders are too narrow.

Solution: Shoulder pads were invented for you. If your facial features are rounded, you'll look better in smaller, softer shoulder pads. If your face is more angular, use larger square or epaulet shoulder pads. Another way to broaden your shoulders is to choose garments with shoulder seams slightly outside your shoulder bones. The same goes for sleeveless dresses: The fabric should end outside your shoulder bones. A cap sleeve also broadens the shoulder.

Problem: My shoulders are too broad.

Solution: Stay away from shoulder pads, boat necklines (they draw the eye across, emphasizing the shoulder line) and details at the shoulder. You'll look great in a V- or scoop-neck with a soft shoulder look, or raglan (loosely fitted) sleeves. Nonfitted sleeve styles (raglan, batwing, kimono) pull the eye inward and down, so they look best on a girl with broad or square shoulders.

Arms

Problem: My arms are too big.

Solution: Avoid sleeves that are tight or clingy.

Problem: My arms are too short.

Solution: A three-quarter sleeve makes the arm and the entire torso appear longer. Cuffs shorten the arm, so avoid cuffs.

Problem: My arms are too long.

Solution: Cuffs shorten the appearance of the arm. A girl with long arms may have trouble finding long sleeves that reach her wrist, but this doesn't have to keep you from buying that outfit you love if you consider adding a cuff to it.

Bust

Problem:　My bust is too large.

Solution:　A short sleeve draws the eye up; if you're large busted, go for short sleeves that end above or below the bustline (rather than right at the bustline). You can also draw attention from your bustline by wearing darker colors on top. Open necklines, long sleeves and loose-fitting clothes with vertical stripes or piping on the bodice will minimize your bustline, too. Avoid tight-fitting tops, breast pockets and high waistbands. Avoid low necklines and high waistlines, which will call attention to your breasts.

Problem:　My bust is too small.

Solution:　If you have a small bustline and you'd like it to appear larger, try wearing textured materials and tweeds, loose-fitting tops with high necklines (turtlenecks and cowl necklines are great), yokes, or bodices with details like pockets, bows, ties, buttons, gathers, pleats or embroidery. You can also enhance your bustline by wearing a bra with padding.

Waistline

Problem:　I'm too short-waisted.

Solution:　A skirt with a yoke around the hips, a dropped waist or no waistband at all will help to lengthen your upper body. A medium-to-narrow belt the same color as your top will have the same effect.

Problem:　My upper torso is too long.

Solution:　An empire waist (high, just under the bustline) or a wide belt the same color and fabric as your skirt will help to shorten a long torso.

Hips

Problem: My hips are too large.

Solution: A long over-blouse with a dropped belt draws attention away from your hips, so they will appear smaller. Gathered skirts, loose pleats, hip pockets and decorative details at the hipline accentuate your hips, so stick with stitched-down or inverted pleats. Wear pants and skirts in deep solid colors. Avoid patterns and light colors on the bottom.

Problem: My hips are too flat.

Solution: If you want to make your hips appear to be more filled out, go for those styles that have pockets and hipline decoration. Gathered skirts and loose pleats also work for you.

Legs

Problem: My legs are very long and gangly looking.

Solution: Wear skirts with a yoke, hemlines at or below the knee, or long pants with pleats and cuffs.

Problem: My legs are too short.

Solution: A short skirt will make your legs appear longer. You can also achieve this effect with a high waistline, cropped pant legs and stockings that match your shoes or skirt.

Feet

Problem: My feet are too big.

Solution: Wear shoes that fit the shape of your foot without adding the appearance of additional length or width. Boots and platform shoes will make your feet look bigger, as will decorations such as buckles, bows and tassels. Darker colors will make your feet appear smaller; whites and pastels always make feet appear larger.

Problem: My feet are too small.

Solution: Wear shoes that fit yet add the illusion of size such as wide heels and thick soles. You can also achieve a larger look with a multi-colored shoe as well as those with fancy decor such as straps, buckles and bows.

Knowing your body and understanding what looks good on you is an important first step in looking great in your clothes. In the following chapter, you'll see just how big an effect color can have on you and your appearance.

15

What Colors Look Best on You?

Vow to be valiant;
resolve to be radiant; determine to be dynamic;
strive to be sincere; aspire to be attuned.

—WILLIAM ARTHUR WARD

Want Tickets to See Ricky Martin?

Wearing the "right" colors can really make a difference. You might be surprised at just *how* much. Think about the last new outfit you bought. Do you think its magic will:

✓ Get you moved to the front of the line for tickets to see Ricky Martin?

✓ Bring out your natural beauty?

✓ Get you an A on an algebra test you haven't studied for?

✓ Get you noticed in a crowd?

✓ Get you a date with Leonardo DiCaprio?

✓ Reduce your stress levels?

✓ Get your parents to advance your allowance?

✓ Make you more self-confident?

✓ Get you voted by your peers as "most likely to succeed"?

✓ Make you feel happier?

✓ Help you identify the kids in your class most likely to get a car when they turn sixteen so you can start sucking up to them?

Well, *okay,* maybe wearing the "right" color won't get you everything you want, but it can make the difference in how you look—and feel! In the questions above, every other one is possible to achieve by wearing the colors that are best suited to you.

Feeling "Blue"? "Green" with Envy? In the "Pink"?

When you forget to study for a test, get a bad grade, and are depressed, do you say, "I'm feeling blue"? When you are jealous because the boy you like asked someone else to the dance, do you say, "I'm green with envy"? Ever hear a cowboy in a Western movie talk about a coward and say, "He's yellow"? When you visit your grandmother does she say, "I'm feeling in the pink today"?

If you think about it, you'll realize that you talk about colors all the time. Color is often the first quality you use to describe something. For example, you don't say, "I bought a cotton shirt" but rather, "I bought a blue cotton shirt." When you talk about a friend, you're likely to say, "She has brown hair and blue eyes."

Because color has so much power over your life, it's important that you know how to use color to your advantage. Psychologists have done studies proving that colors can do things like cheer people up (red seems to make people happy), calm people down (pink is soothing). Did you know that some prisons actually paint their walls pink to try to calm down the inmates? Hospitals often paint rooms green because it is a "healing" color, and blue appears to help people stay focused on a task, to concentrate harder.

What Is _Your_ Favorite Color?

What is your favorite color? Do you have a lot of clothes in that color? Do you buy things like backpacks and book covers in that color? My friend is a pink freak. Everything she owns is pink. She painted her bedroom furniture pink. She has pink sheets and blankets. She has a pink slipcover over the seat of her car. And of course, the car has a bumper sticker that says THINK PINK! We tease her about her obsession, but Keesha just shrugs and says, "Pink makes me happy."

What color makes you happy?

How Colors Can Make You Prettier

Colors can do more than make you feel good; they can make you look good. You probably already know that certain colors complement your face, while other colors make you look washed-out or sallow. When you wear your bright-turquoise silk shirt, do people tell you that you're looking especially pretty that day? I have an aquamarine sweater that is very bright and cheerful. Whenever I wear it, my girlfriends tell me that I'm "looking happy." It's just that the sweater is really my color and makes me feel good. Why is that?

To know which colors can help you look prettier, you need to understand a little bit about colors themselves. I was at the mall one day, looking for a new dress to wear to a very special upcoming party. I was a senior in high school at the time. The salesclerk asked me what I had in mind, and I said, "I'd like something in a really pretty color. I know all my friends will be in black dresses, but I don't want to wear black. I feel better in earth-tone colors." The clerk smiled and said, "Oh, you must be an autumn girl."

Autumn girl? I had never heard that term before. I asked the clerk what she meant, and she and I got into a really interesting discussion about "having your colors done." Have you ever heard that expression? Have you ever had your "colors done"?

The System of Seasons

The system of seasons is about the shades each of us look best in based upon our hair and eye coloring and the tone of our skin. For example, a "spring" girl is usually a blonde with very light skin. She probably has blue or hazel eyes. This coloring makes her look nice in colors like apricot, coral, red, yellow and aqua. My good friend Sarah is a spring, as is my mother. My friends Randee and Nghin, are autumn girls, like me. Autumn girls have gray-green or brown eyes, chestnut hair, or red hair (from auburn to coppery red to "carrot top"), and skin with a yellowish tinge. Autumn girls look great in earth tones, like brown, golds and beiges, but not so great in deep blues. When Sarah dyed her hair black and began wearing a much darker makeup, she looked completely different when wearing colors like apricot or yellow. Normally these soft colors created a halo around her and when she dyed her hair black, the colors created an almost stark appearance. Of course, you can wear whatever color you like. And you should. The advantage of knowing your "season" is that you can complement the color of your hair, eyes and skin tone—this is a real bonus in looking your very best, maybe even in *feeling* your very best.

What season are you? Below is a chart to help you identify your season, as well as highlight those colors that look best on you.

Season	Hair	Eyes	Skin	Best Colors
SPRING	light	light	fair	clear, warm, crisp colors: pink, apricot, salmon, coral, gold
SUMMER	light	light	rosy	pastels, neutrals, rose, most blues, lavender
AUTUMN	reddish	hazel	golden	muted or clear earth tones: teal, periwinkle, gold, oyster white
WINTER	dark	dark	olive and dark	clear, cool colors; true red, turquoise, navy blue, black, pure white

Are You a Spring, Summer, Autumn or Winter Girl?

Each of the following three pages has a picture of a girl who represents the season described on the page. There are, of course, some variations, but for the most part, these seasonal recommendations ring true. My goal is to help you understand the idea that certain colors work best for some girls, but may not necessarily look as vibrant and appealing on others. The goal is to use this knowledge of your hair, eyes and skin tone to select those colors that are really special for you. You might also want to put this information to the test: Think about the girls at school who always seem so well-dressed, so put-together. Can you identify which seasons they are? Do they look better in some colors than in others? Let's take a look at the "four seasons."

What's Fresh for Spring Girls

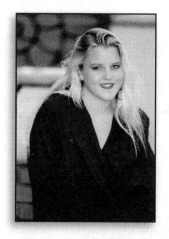

My friend Tawny Flippen [see photo here and color-plate 1] is a typical Spring, with golden hair tones, blue eyes and peachy skin tone. Spring girls have a wide array to choose from. If you are a Spring, you look pretty in apricot, salmon, coral and pink—but rose and mauve are not so good on a Spring. Any light orange, bright coral or orange-red looks good on you. Clear red is good, but avoid a red with a bluish tint and colors that are muted. You can wear yellow, yellow-green, medium and bright greens, many shades of aqua and turquoise, teal and peacock blue, light true blue, periwinkle blue and medium violet. Your best white is creamy ivory, and you wear beige and camel well. Clear golds, rusts and browns from golden tan to chocolate also look good on you. You can wear a light yellowish-gray, but rarely a true gray. A light, clear navy blue or black is good. Spring's colors are clear, bright or delicate with yellow undertones as you can see by the color chart on colorplate 5.

What's Hot for Summer Girls

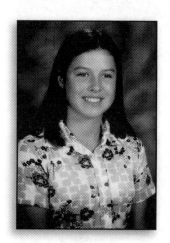

Renee Moreno [see photo here and colorplate 2] is a typical Summer: ash hair, gray-blue eyes and a rosy complexion. If you are a Summer girl, you look awesome in pastels and soft neutral colors. Avoid sharp contrasts in colors, since they will leave you looking washed out. Blues were made for you, soft but ranging from light to deep, including aqua and blues with a pinkish cast, all the way to mauve and orchid, and even fuchsia, plum, burgundy and raspberry with a powdered finish. You look superb in soft pinks and roses, and your browns and beiges should have a rose undertone. Your navy should have a gray cast to it, keeping it soft. Red, gray and green tempered with a hint of blue are good for you. Except for a light lemon color, yellows and golds are best avoided, as are all colors with yellow undertones. You should also stay away from black, and your white should be very soft. Summer's colors are soft and cool with blue undertones as you can see from the color chart on colorplate 6.

The Shades of Autumn Girls

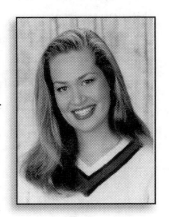

My natural coloring [see photo here and colorplate 3] is that of a typical Autumn: warm brown hair with highlights of red or blonde, hazel eyes and golden skin. If you're an Autumn girl, you have a lot of colors to choose from. You can wear either muted or clear tones. You wear all earth tones well—browns, golds, yellows, greens, oranges and orange-reds. Blues are the area where you have the least adaptability, so stick to strong and muted turquoise, and teal and deep periwinkle. You look pretty in oyster white, a white with a beige tone. You look good in all beiges except rosy beige and gray-beige. Black, navy, gray, pink and colors with blue undertones are not for you. If you are an Autumn girl like me, our best colors are those that are stronger than Spring's and have gold or orange overtones, as shown on the color chart on colorplate 7.

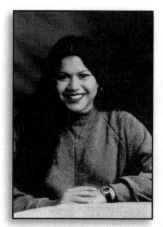

What's Cool for Winter Girls

Lena Arceo [see photo here and colorplate 4] is a typical Winter girl: dark hair and eyes, beige, tan, olive or dark skin. Winter girls look best in clear colors with sharp contrasts. The key is to keep your colors clear and vivid and to avoid anything with a yellowish cast. Your colors are strong, and solids are better for you than prints, especially near your face. You shine in icy colors (so pale you'd almost think they were white). Stay away from muted tones and powdered pastels. Clear reds and greens, blues and turquoises, all the bluish shades of pink, and purples were made for you. You wear navy and burgundy well. You look fabulous in true white, true black and true grays from light to charcoal. Beiges are not great for you, but you can wear a clear taupe (gray-beige). You can get away with a clear, bright lemon yellow, but stay away from golden yellow, gold and golden brown. Remember: Winter's colors are vivid, clear or icy with blue undertones. The color chart on colorplate 8 shows colors that are all yours.

Shop with Your Colors in Mind —And in Hand

If this is your first introduction to wearing the colors that look best on you, it can seem like a lot of trouble. But once you see and feel the difference a certain color makes, you will get better and better at selecting clothing with your best colors in mind.

Using your newfound information, go back again to your Clothing Inventory [see chapter 13]. Thinking about the colors that work best with your hair and eye coloring and your skin tone, would you say that most of the clothes in your wardrobe are in the colors that best complement you? If you look great in bright colors but not so great in pastels, a closet full of pastels tells you that it's time to shop with your color chart in hand.

Once you have a better idea of what colors look best on you, you'll want to buy clothes in those colors. So when you go shopping, take along the page from this book that shows your best colors. You may even want to get swatches of your colors. These are professional kits that show the colors of each season not only on paper, but in actual fabrics. You can buy these in some department stores and fabric stores. And if you get your "colors done" by someone who has been specially trained (check with a salesclerk at your department stores), as a rule, that person will give you a swatch of your preferred colors as a courtesy.

Short of that, go to a fabric store with two of your good friends. Hold up different fabrics close to your face, and ask your friends to tell you which colors make you look your prettiest. Tell your friends to concentrate on your face, not on the fabric. A fabric store is a wonderful place to "do your colors" because of the wide variety of shades and hues of material.

Knowing which colors don't work for you can save you a lot of time and—even more importantly—money. What if you saw an adorable little dress and just had to have it? You might buy it even without trying it on if you were in a hurry—only to get home and realize that though the cut and style are okay, there's something about the color that just doesn't work for you. Had you known that earth colors were not good for you, you could have passed on buying it in the first place. Just because the mannequin with the black hair, dark eyes and glossy red lip color looked spectacular in that bright-red dress, if you have blue eyes and ash brown hair, it may not look as hot on you as you had hoped. Again, certain colors and certain styles look better on us than others do. It's why the mannequins come equipped with an assortment of wig colors, and their eyes and lips are often painted over to bring out the best in the fabric, color and fashion being displayed!

Here's another helpful suggestion: Now that you have an idea of how colors and seasons work, try to get help from a salesperson who shares your season. She'll be much better at spotting the right colors for you. This is especially important if you shop with a friend of a different season, as she will naturally (and unconsciously) tend to suggest colors that would look better on her.

A Dose of Dashing Dazzle

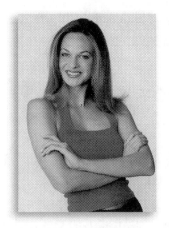

I have one final comment on the power of colors. My high school's colors were red and white. Every Friday was school spirit day, and everyone was supposed to wear red and white. One girl in school always wore the same red and white that the rest of us did, but for some reason, while the rest of us looked liked clones, she always stood apart from us, and managed to look very chic. It wasn't until I was talking about this girl, Kim, with my mom, that I realized what was different. If Kim wore a red T-shirt, she would have the collar of a blue-rimmed T-shirt showing just a tad around the neck area. Blue was Kim's color; next to her face, it looked great. If Kim wore a red sweater, she would have a great scarf wrapped around her neck, again drawing attention away from the huge red sweatshirt that made us all look like giant apples. It was just those little finishing touches, a small dash of dazzling colors that did the most to enhance Kim's natural beauty, that made her always look so great, so put-together.

With a little thought, you can dress to suit your body type, your coloring, your personality and your mood. The next chapter will show you how you can accessorize—add bracelets, earrings, scarves and necklaces as Kim did in the example above—to add pizzazz to the way you look, as well as to change the look of your outfit.

16

It's the Little Things That Count: Accessories

*Remember the most beautiful
things in the world are the most useless;
peacocks and lilies, for instance.*

—JOHN RUSKIN

Do You Wear Your Boyfriend's Ring on a Chain?

Carrie did. All through our senior year, my friend Carrie wore her boyfriend's ring on a chain around her neck. It was a large silver ring and she wore it all the time. When she was wearing sweatshirts and other casual clothes, it hung on a long, heavy silver chain—it looked really cool. When she wore it with her black velour floor-length prom dress, the ring hung on a shorter, winding silver chain that sparkled—it looked elegant. When she wore a wide-lapel, very formal business suit to an important job interview, she added a scarf that matched her suit perfectly, and knotted the scarf using her boyfriend's ring as a tie—it looked sophisticated. Accessories are like that. One piece can dress up one outfit and then, with just a little imagination, the same piece can look fantastic in an entirely different way with a completely different outfit. It can add to the beauty of whatever outfit you are wearing.

For Better or for Worse

Accessories add, or detract from, style. Earrings, bracelets, necklaces, scarves, belts, even pins can change the look of your outfit for better or for worse. Maybe you have a friend who always wears scarves. Scarves often look great with feminine outfits but may look out of place with a sweatshirt and sweatpants.

Your accessories should complement, rather than demolish, what you're wearing. They should add that extra little touch that makes an outfit memorable, exciting and fun. I was at the mall recently and my eyes were instantly drawn to a beautiful African-American woman, perhaps college age, who was wearing black slacks, black boots, and a black sweater offset by a very large ornate pair of silver and turquoise earrings. The earrings were so attention-getting that you couldn't help but notice her. The earrings really worked for her, most especially against the all-black background of her outfit. It was an awesome look, and made her striking. Make your accessories work for you.

What types of accessories do you have in your closet and drawers? Go back to your Clothing Inventory in chapter 13. What accessories did you list? You probably had all sorts of jewelry, like rings, necklaces and bracelets. Maybe you had some scarves, a hat or two, and some earrings. Look over your comments. Did you occasionally jot a note like, "Drab. Needs some pizzazz," or "Doesn't quite work"? If a little something is missing, it just might be the right accessories.

Here are some ways you can add a touch of beauty and zest to your appearance.

Why Knot Add Some Class with Scarves?

One easy, quick and classy way to accessorize is by using scarves. Scarves can be as simple as a red paisley bandanna (the kind the cowboys wore around their necks) or as sophisticated as a large silk rectangle with fringe. My friend Frankie Welch, of Frankie Welch Designs, has created over four thousand scarves, many of which have been designed specifically for corporations, museums and universities. She has created really interesting scarves for individuals who have commissioned her designs, including seven American presidents and their first ladies [see colorplates 40–45]. I think having a scarf designed especially for yourself is pretty cool! It's definitely on my "wish list"! (Frankie is currently designing a Taste Berries for Teens scarf!)

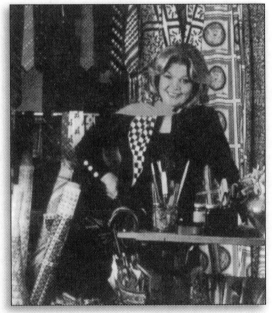

Frankie Welch

Frankie, who has been a media spokesperson for the textile industry, says you're never too young to start a scarf collection. "Look for beautiful, colorful scarves," Frankie advises. "Buy them on sale, and when you're tired of wearing one, store it away. It will always be good. A classic scarf will always be in style. Look for a beautiful scarf. Designs remain the same, so even if you get tired of it for one season, you will love it a year from now. If your scarf is beginning to show wear, use it for a pocket square. You can also frame it to give color to a room."

Four Nifty Ways
to Add Jazz with a Scarf

What are some of the things you personally can do with scarves? Here's just a short list; you can probably think of a dozen more points yourself.

- The right scarf adds color and dresses up a plain pair of jeans or slacks and a plain blouse or sweater. A scarf can give the whole outfit a new look. Depending on the colors and fabrics, a scarf can make an outfit more sophisticated, more trendy, more glamorous, more playful—more alive.

- A scarf tied around a ponytail makes an interesting "new" hairstyle and can add a touch of color to an otherwise plain or one-colored outfit. You may want to wrap your entire head in the scarf, turban style. (A scarf can also be used on that "should have washed my hair but didn't" hairstyle, whether to cover it up or pull it into a great decorated ponytail!)

- Suppose you're having one of those days where you feel blasé and no outfit looks just right. Wrap a small brightly colored scarf around your wrist, tie in a small bow and watch all the attention and compliments you get. It will make you feel more lighthearted and fun, and it's sure to help you lighten up!

- A scarf makes a great belt. No matter how many belts you have, there is always that one outfit for which you can't find the perfect belt. All your belts are the wrong color or wrong style, but you really think a belt will finish the outfit just right. If you have a scarf in the right color, use it as a belt instead.

From Tiaras to Tongue Studs

From tiaras to tongue studs, jewelry advertises your style. Some girls love large, funky pieces of jewelry. Others like dainty, delicate pieces. Some wear bracelets; others make a statement with their watches. Of the pieces you listed on your Clothing Inventory, how many of those do you really wear? How have your tastes in jewelry changed as you've matured? Maybe when you were a little girl you wore your Barbie necklace constantly, but today you'd rather kiss your geeky cousin than be seen wearing it.

If you're like most teens, you have a box of jewelry that you haven't worn in ages. How do you decide what jewelry you want to keep? How can you use jewelry to define your style and compliment what you are wearing and flatter your appearance? Here are a few suggestions.

- Use jewelry to draw attention. I have a good friend, Maria, who has the most gorgeous hands, with long slender fingers. She keeps her nails absolutely perfect and calls attention to her hands by wearing pretty and interesting jewelry. Nearly every day Maria wears some different ring or bracelet. We all look forward to seeing her jewelry and can't help but notice her beautiful hands.

- Be trendy. Jewelry has fads and trends, just like everything else. In the 1960s, there were so-called "mood rings," rings that supposedly changed color to indicate your mood. In the 1970s, everyone wore peace symbols. In the 1980s, there were Slappers, the little bracelets that you slapped on around your wrist. The 1990s brought wrist beads for health, wealth, love, friendship, prosperity and more. Trendy jewelry doesn't have to be expensive and it can show that you are "with it." The clip art that is the rage right now is cute and fun and is a good way to add a little color and style without spending much money. Don't feel like you need to follow every fad, but updating yourself now and then can be hip—and fun.

- Choose jewelry that works for you. If you are a petite girl, wearing huge jewelry can be overpowering. You don't want people to say, "The jewelry is wearing her," rather than, "She's wearing the jewelry." Experiment with different pieces in the store, looking in a mirror to see how the jewelry looks on you before buying it.

- Match jewelry to your mood. There are days when you wake up and you are in a lighthearted, fun mood. Great! Wear a silly piece of jewelry that makes everyone smile. I personally have kept (this is so embarrassing!) some of the blue Smurfs jewelry I had when I was a little girl. On days when I'm feeling totally silly, I wear a Smurfs necklace. I love it because it matches my mood. Sometimes, on those days when I'm a grouch, I wear it to remind myself to lighten up.

- Match jewelry to the occasion. You don't wear a tiara with jeans and a flannel shirt! And you don't wear a watch with a thick leather band when you're wearing a silk dress.

- Have a "serious" piece for nice occasions—and to add a touch of class to others. Do you have a nice piece that you use when you dress up? My serious piece was a pearl ring. Whenever I wore my pearl ring, not only did I feel dressed up, it looked classy. On days when I was feeling plain, I didn't feel plain when I put it on; instead I felt rather "special." Maybe you have a nice piece of good jewelry, like a class ring, a gold necklace or a silver bracelet, and you wear it constantly. The good thing about a nice piece of jewelry is that it won't go out of style, you can wear it with everything and it lasts for years.

- Use jewelry to display a special interest. The classic example of this is your class ring. You proudly wear a class ring to show your school spirit. Maybe you have a necklace from a club, or a charm bracelet with special amulets from places you've visited. Anything that you are proud of helps define who you are.

- Make jewelry your trademark. Your "style" of accessories defines your style and becomes a trademark of sorts. One of the first people who comes to mind for me is Serena Williams, the seventeen-year-old tennis champion. The world is so used to seeing her show up on the courts with the beads in her hair that if she didn't wear them in her hair one day, we might not even recognize her! The beaded hair is her trademark—well, of course, the beads and all her trophies! Another person who comes to mind is my friend Olana, who is a figure skater. Every day at the rink, she wears the same basic black bodysuit. She got pretty tired of this outfit, and decided to start brightening it up with pins. Every day she wore a different pin. Some of the pins were silly; some were really nice. She had fun finding unusual pins at swap meets and garage sales. And the rest of us found that we were always keeping an eye out for pins for Olana as well.

- Use an unusual piece of jewelry as a conversation piece. Are you shy? All of us get a little nervous in new situations, like meeting a sweetheart's parents or going to a new school. Everyone stands around, wanting to talk to the others, but not wanting to make the first move. If you wear some unusual piece of jewelry, people feel like they can come up to you and comment on it, and that breaks the ice. I have a pair of silvery earrings that look like birds, and the wings flap when I move my head. (Yeah, I know they sound weird, but they really are cute.) Everyone, both girls and boys, comes up to me and compliments me on them, and asks me where I got them.

Are You Considering Body Piercing or a Tattoo?

Sixteen-year-old Kimmie Jennings works at a little bookstore that I visit frequently. Kimmie is friendly and outgoing, an honors student and an accomplished tennis player. When I came into the bookstore one day last week, the first thing Kimmie said when she saw me was, "Look at this! Look at this!" Pointing to her newly pierced eyebrow, she added, "Over the top! Isn't it?" and took a few steps closer to me so she could show off the small silver earring. "What'd your mom have to say about it?" I asked, having heard Kimmie on occasion talk about her "mother and her rules."

"Oh, it took me months to talk her into it," Kimmie replied, then added, "Once she agreed, well, I admit I got a little scared, but I wasn't about to back out! All my friends have their eyebrows pierced—or their tongues, or their noses, or their belly buttons—or any combination of them."

There was a time when a pierced eyebrow, tongue, nose or navel was reserved for kids who were social rebels making a statement. But that's just not the case anymore. Many teens have body piercing, even tattoos. If you're considering such a piercing, you'll definitely want to make sure you get your parents' permission. It's an unregulated business for the most part, so no one really even knows how common body-piercing infections are—which is one reason you want to enlist your parents' support: You want to watch out for the chance of infections, and your parents can help you find the right place to have your piercing done. The right place means one where the procedure is done with sterilization and the correct metals (such as surgical steel or gold). Here are some other things you'll want to consider:

- Health-care professionals report that body piercing and tattooing can cause infections (especially a pierced eyebrow since it's the area most likely to be touched repeatedly throughout the day).
- Piercing the eyebrow causes the skin around the eye to stretch and droop.
- Dentists report tongue jewelry is the leading cause of chipped teeth.
- Tongue piercing can cause problems with chewing your food, numbness in your tongue resulting in being unable to speak clearly, as well as permanent nerve damage.
- There is the risk of being infected with hepatitis B and C, especially in cases of self-piercing and sharing instruments.
- Navel piercing is often irritated by clothing. Additionally, there are frequent reports that the skin can heal over on the navel and cover the whole ring—which means that the skin will have to be lanced so the ring can be removed.

- Aside from the risk of local infection of the skin, there is also the risk of contact dermatitis (itchy, scaly rash when the skin reacts to jewelry) and keloid formations (overgrowth of scar tissue).

Perhaps you've seen the commercial where one guy says to another, "My daughter is hounding me about getting a tattoo. What do you think about tattoos?" The other guy shrugs and says, "My father had a tattoo," to which the first guy replies, "But did your mother?" It's a good point. Tattooing is less preferable than body piercing because though it carries all the same risks, it's a permanent procedure. That intricate dainty butterfly or wildflower the length of your leg, or the barbed wire around your arm or ankle will be there for the rest of your life (unless you have it surgically removed or with a laser). My suggestion is if you are considering a tattoo or piercing think three times first.

If you really want the look or the body art, a great alternative is temporary paste-on tattoos. You can find them in a wide variety of beautiful artwork, and they can give you the same look, but since they aren't permanent you won't be answering your future grandchildren's questions about them. Besides that, there's no risk of infection and you'll save yourself a lot of money.

Swapping Instead of Shopping: Accessories Exchange

Your allowance or part-time job paycheck doesn't go very far when you hit the mall. It's easy to spend an entire month's income on one sweater or that really great bikini. If you are spending most of your money on clothes, you may not feel as if you have a cent to spare for accessories. That's where friends come to your rescue.

It may be hard to borrow clothes from friends (although I'm willing to bet you try!). Not everyone can wear the same size (I know: I'm tall and most of my short girlfriends' clothes don't fit me). And we certainly don't all like the same styles. Besides, sometimes people are a little nervous about lending out clothes. I have a leather jacket that I won't lend to anyone, even to my best friend, because I know I could never replace it if it were lost. But accessories are something else entirely.

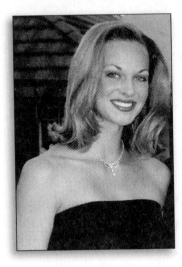

You probably have a dozen pieces of jewelry in your drawers that you hardly wear, and a few scarves that have dust on them. Call your friends and schedule an accessories exchange. You can either permanently swap jewelry and scarves, or just borrow items from each other. Sometimes you can't really tell whether you like big jewelry or smaller jewelry until you've worn the piece for a while. My friend Mike bought a big, thick, heavy silver necklace. He thought it looked macho and wore it proudly—for about a day. Then he complained about how heavy the necklace was, how it caught in his clothes, and how he just couldn't stand it. I agreed to go with him to exchange the necklace. He got a lighter one and is much happier. But the point is, he had to go through all that fuss. If you borrow jewelry and accessories from your friends, you can try various pieces at home without having to put out any money. A word to the wise: Always return the things you borrow. Not only is it unfair not to, but you can lose a good friend if you take goodwill too far. Be courteous.

Of course, maybe your whole goal is not to prevent shopping, but to go shopping as much as possible. In that case, it's important you know how to be a good shopper, and the next chapter can help you become just that!

17

Shopping, Shopping, Shopping, Shopping, Shopping

*Every small task of everyday life is
part of the total harmony
of the universe.*

—St. Theresa of Lisieux

Get Ready, Get Set, Shop!

If you were going to take a final exam, you would do your homework and put in time studying, correct? If you were going to run a marathon, you would prepare by training for weeks, and then stretching just before starting, right? Smart people plan ahead for activities. Shopping (my own personal favorite activity!) also requires planning and homework.

A wise shopper knows what styles and colors work best for her. She knows how to distinguish what she needs from what she wants. If you are prepared before you head out, you won't find yourself toting several bags home from the mall only to realize you didn't really need the sweater you bought, or that you should have invested in a skirt to go with the sweater instead of allowing yourself to be swept off your feet by that cute little number that didn't go with anything you owned. And, what about that pair of shoes the salesman said "would stretch," only you can't bear to wear them long enough for them to do so? Definitely not a good buy!

You can't blame yourself entirely. Everything conspires to make you spend your money. Stores know how to make their products incredibly tempting to you. Companies hire decorators who know just how to arrange the displays to catch your eye with the latest trends, and they make certain to assure you that you can't live without their goods. (Not to mention the pressure you feel at the urging of your friend who already happens to own a pair of five-inch, rhinestone-studded, patent-leather platform shoes that lace up to the knees, and has threatened that the friendship between the two of you depends on your owning a pair, too. You've seen her walk around her room in them, they're eye-catching all right, but you're not convinced you could go out of the house with them let alone stay upright throughout the day!) Everyone at the store is looking to sell you something—that's the business they are in. It's up to you to make sure that you aren't foolish or gullible and that you make the best use of your shopping time and money!

Shop Smarter, Not Harder

How can you be a smart shopper, making the best choices? As you browse through the racks of clothes, ask yourself the following questions:

Is It a Wise Buy?

So there you are, walking past the store and in the window you see this very incredible jacket with a gorgeous blazing-red lining. The colors are just amazing, more dazzling than anything you've ever seen; best of all, the jacket is marked down 35 percent. Ten minutes later, the jacket is in your bag! Two hours later, you're home staring at yourself in the mirror, thinking, "Why did I buy this? I already have a jacket that's a lot more practical, and besides, I live in Orlando, Florida; I'll almost never wear something this hot and heavy."

Like many of us, you were attracted by the sales price. Sure, a good shopper should take advantage of sales, but don't let a good price seduce you into buying something you won't wear. Remember, a sale item is no bargain if you don't have anything to wear it with in the end (especially if you're unlikely to spend the money to buy whatever else it needs in order to be a complete outfit). It's also anything but a bargain if it doesn't make you look good. You may have saved $17.96 on that jacket, but if you never wear it, it becomes a very expensive hanger ornament in your closet!

Is It a Good Fit?

The second question you need to ask yourself when you are thinking of buying clothing is whether it fits you well. You should be able to pinch between one and two inches of fabric around your torso, arms and legs. Don't get into the habit of saying, "I'm always a size ten (or four, or fourteen, or whatever)." Sizes vary a lot from designer to designer, and from product to product. I have a good friend who tells me she has clothes in sizes six, eight and ten. She's a smart shopper who knows to go for the fit rather than the size on the label. Try everything on, especially those items purchased where "all sales are final."

Don't just stand in front of the mirror, admiring the beauty of the fabric and design of what you have on. Move around a little in the clothes and see how they work for you. Sleeves with seams narrower than your shoulder bones and cuffs that ride up your arm when you bend your elbow will make you look like you borrowed your little sister's clothes. Jacket sleeves should reveal about a half inch of your blouse sleeve at the wrist. Remember to try your jackets on over your clothes, to make sure they have no pull across the back or the front when you button them. Garments that gap between the buttons or pull across the back when you reach out or fold your arms in front of you are just too small. Your jeans and slacks should break at the top of your shoes, not be so long you step on them. Pockets should stay closed, and pleats and darts should lie flat. A skirt that rides up when you sit down or pants and skirts so tight you can see panty lines are unappealing. I think it looks natural for a skirt to curve in a little bit, but if it hugs the hips too tightly you should go for the next-larger size.

And let's not forget that it's possible to buy clothes that are too big as well. Sure, the baggy look can be stylish sometimes; it's a fad that comes and goes. For a while, everyone wore jeans that were so large they practically fell off the hips, and sweatshirts that could have housed a family of four and had room left over for their neighbors! It's fun to wear the occasionally funky, fashionable outfit, just to make a statement. And of course, it's always wise to go for clothes that compliment your self-confidence and comfort.

Is It Easy to Care For?

Quick: Name three things you'd rather do than spend an afternoon ironing. Here's my list:

- ✓ Hang out with my friends and boyfriend.
- ✓ Work out.
- ✓ Wash the windows at my apartment.

For most of us, ironing is not a favorite activity. Therefore, a smart shopper thinks about fabric care before she buys the item. Notice how on Sasha's inventory she cites two items she doesn't like because of the way they look.

It just so happens that in her case, both garments are linen, a fabric that takes a lot of care. If you don't want to iron your clothing, the logical thing to do is to look for wrinkle-free clothes. You can identify fabric that won't wrinkle easily by crushing a handful of the fabric and squeezing it tightly. When you let go, notice whether the fabric stays wrinkled or smoothes out easily. If the wrinkles stay in, the garment will probably need a lot of ironing. In addition, the piece may look wrinkled ten minutes after you've ironed it. I hardly ever wear one of my favorite shirts because it wrinkles so quickly. I can iron it, get in the car, put on my seat belt—and within minutes my shirt is all wrinkled again. That's very frustrating! However, if something does wrinkle a little bit, don't despair. You can still avoid some ironing by taking your clothes out of the dryer (assuming they are washable and don't require dry cleaning) as soon as they are dry (or even slightly damp) and hanging them up in your closet immediately. If you leave them tossed in a heap on your bed, the wrinkles will be set in, and they'll be hard to get out even with an iron.

Fabrics such as linen, rayon or silk wrinkle easily, whereas polished cotton, fleece or wool do not. Look back over your Clothing Inventory. Do any of the reasons for not liking an item have to do with the fabric always looking messy or unkempt?

And what about dry cleaning? Some clothes can't be washed but have to be dry cleaned, which can get expensive. Can you afford to have your clothes dry cleaned? Will your parents make you pay for the dry cleaning out of your hard-earned allowance or paycheck? Dry cleaning in effect makes the price of the item higher than you originally thought. Say for example you spent $30 on a nice blouse. If you have to pay $5 to get it cleaned every time you wear it, in six months or so, the price of the blouse has been doubled. If the shirt had cost $60 when you saw it in the store, would you have bought it in the first place? Look at the labels on the clothing, and see whether they say *Dry Clean Only*. If they do, think really hard about whether you want to buy that item.

(Of course, some things, like prom dresses or really good jackets that you wear only on special occasions, have to be dry cleaned. That's okay, because you won't be wearing them often.)

Is It a Necessary Purchase?

When you go out to a buffet dinner with your folks, you probably look at all those great gooey desserts and say to your mom, "I'd like that and that and that, and ooooh yeah, I would really like that!" You both laugh, but of course you don't end up chowing down every single dessert. Just because you want something doesn't mean you need it. The same thing is true for clothing. You may want every shirt you see on the rack, but do you need them all?

Every time you think about buying something, stop and ask yourself, "Is it necessary? Do I really need this item, or do I just want it?" When you already have five black T-shirts, do you want to buy a sixth one just because it has a designer's name on the front? If you have three denim jackets, do you need to spend more money on another simply because the buttons on it are cute? One way I have learned to identify what I want versus what I need is through using my Clothing Inventory. This is another way you can make your Clothing Inventory work for you.

Dressing for Success, Not Excess

A closet of clothes that work together to bring out the best in you doesn't happen by accident. It takes work and planning to make your wardrobe all you need it to be. This is where your Clothing Inventory is useful. A Clothing Inventory can help you in three important ways.

1. *It identifies what you already have in your closet and drawers, so you don't buy the same thing.* I remember my girlfriend Marcy telling me one day, "I can't believe it. I was at the store and I spent all my money on this absolutely great belt, which I loved. Then I got home and put it on my belt rack—right next to one that was almost identical. And worst of all, it was on sale and can't be returned. A Clothing Inventory identifies pieces you already have so you don't buy similar things.

2. *It identifies what you need.* Maybe you forgot that you spilled a cranberry smoothie down the front of your favorite white blouse, thereby turning it into a car-wash rag. And your next-favorite blouse is way too small, thanks to that recent growth spurt. You don't want to wait until five minutes before a pep-squad photo session to find out you don't have the white shirt that you need for the group picture. A Clothing Inventory keeps you up-to-date on what things you need to replace.

3. *It identifies what you can match.* A smart shopper makes the most of her clothing dollar by buying items that work together. What good does it do you to buy that great skirt if you don't have something that works with it? When you buy something that has no "mate" (something to wear along with it), one of two things happens. Either you never wear the new piece, relegating it to the back of your closet, or you go back to the store and spend yet more money on something to match the new piece.

It's What You Do with What You've Got

You've probably seen the commercials in which someone has just won a World Cup soccer match or the Super Bowl. The camera focuses on the person, who is asked, "What are you going to do now?" The person yells, *"I'm going to Disneyland!"* Well, I have a fantasy like that, but it doesn't involve Disneyland. I dream that someday I am going to win 20 million dollars in the lottery. The newscaster is going to say, "You've just won 20 million dollars! What are you going to do now?" I'm going to grin and shout back, *"I'm going to Bloomingdale's!"*

Alas, I haven't won the lottery yet, but when it comes to clothes, the good news is, I don't have to. The key is to make the most of what you've got already. If you shop wisely, you should be able to create at least thirty different looks with as few as ten to fifteen pieces of clothing.

The secret is to coordinate shapes and colors to create complementary outfits using a minimum of basic pieces. This technique will save you money, time and the headache of wondering what you're going to wear.

Following a Master Plan

Let me introduce you to the master plan. Here are the basic pieces you will need to get in order to have a wardrobe that is ample enough to take you anywhere you need to be—from hanging at the mall with your friends, to going on a once-in-a-lifetime date with the guy of your dreams, to suffering through those intimidating job or college interviews.

- A jacket or two: Choose a jacket in a classic style with matching buttons or no buttons at all. The fabric can be natural or a high-quality synthetic, in colors that bring out the best in you. If necessary, have it tailored (sleeves shortened or lengthened, for example) to suit your shape. If you choose a second jacket, select a complementary color to the skirts and pants you already have or intend to buy.

- Two skirts: You need a short straight skirt and a fuller skirt of whatever length best flatters your figure. Each should be in colors to complement both jackets. For example, if you have a navy-blue jacket, you might have a matching navy-blue skirt, but also a white skirt or a camel-colored skirt.

- Pants: Select pants to fit your figure in a solid neutral color that goes with your jackets. Your pants should be of a quality fabric, that is made well enough to handle the wear and tear of busy teen life. The pants may also need to be hemmed, and you may want to leave some length of fabric to let the hem down as you grow taller.

- Three blouses: Every girl's wardrobe should have a simple white, off-white or ivory-colored blouse, another everyday blouse in a print or solid color with front buttons (long enough to be used as an over-blouse) and a dressier blouse in a solid color. Coordinate the colors and styles to go with your skirts, pants and jackets.

- Two sweaters and/or knit tops: A cardigan sweater can work as a jacket or a blouse. Choose your other sweater or knit top with a neckline that suits you. Both sweaters should be in plain colors to complement your skirts, pants and jackets. For summertime, a short-sleeved cotton knit is good.

- One or two dresses: Your first dress should have long sleeves and be in a solid color in a simple style that can be dressed up for evening wear. Select a weight appropriate for the season of the year. A second dress can be a one- or two-piece in a print or pattern. For both, choose colors that look good with your jackets.

- Evening dress and skirt or pants: Choose a dressy fabric (satin, brocade or velvet, for example) for your evening clothes. It's a good idea to select a two-piece dress for versatility, and coordinate the colors so you can wear the top with your evening skirt or pants.

- Coat: Depending on where you live, you may need a heavy coat or just a light one. Select a neutral color that will go with everything you wear.

The lines should be simple, with matching buttons. Choose a quality fabric and a style to flatter your body type.

Fads, Fashion and "Extreme Edge" Trends

When you were going through your closet and drawers to make your Clothing Inventory, did you come across a few pieces of clothing that are so-o-o outdated they make you grimace? If you're like me, you have some clothes that you thought you absolutely couldn't live without—and now you wouldn't be seen dead wearing! I have one skirt made out of fake fur in a cow pattern, white with big black blotches. I remember paying an outrageous amount of money for it (goaded on by my best friend who said, "That is so cool, Jen, so with it!") I wore the skirt exactly once, and after the ribbing I took from wearing that gaudy thing, I then buried it in the back of my closet. What a waste of money that was.

Obviously, clothing fads change quite often. Sure, it's fun to buy an occasional fad outfit, something wild and crazy, but you don't want a closet filled with only the latest fashions. What happens when the latest fashion becomes yesterday's news? You'll be back to staring at your closet and moaning that you have nothing to wear.

Choose clothes that are comfortable, and ones that fit your day-to-day activities—your lifestyle. This doesn't mean you shouldn't keep up with the style and be trendy. But before you buy that expensive pair of five-inch buffalo boots, clomping the cutting edge of fashion, ask yourself how often you would actually wear them. If the answer is, "oh, once or twice," pass on the boots, even if they did look "totally cool" on your favorite rock diva. Skousers, bindis and flares that are "in" this month are sure to look naff (unfashionable) three months from now. And do you want to still be paying your mom or dad back for the money you borrowed to buy clothes you never wear anymore?

In summary, a wise shopper (that's you!) recognizes three things:

✓ What types of clothes look good on her.

✓ What clothing she already has and how to make the most outfits and different looks from the fewest pieces.

✓ How to spend her clothing money wisely to fill in gaps in her wardrobe and still have some money left over for fun.

Making Your Wish/Want/Need List!

You've already done the hard part of the Clothing Inventory—going through everything to decide what you have and what condition it is in. Now you get to reward yourself with the fun part of the task—listing what you need to buy. Fill in the following chart. Make several copies of it. I suggest you keep one copy in your wallet (or your mom's wallet, if she'll be the one whipping out the credit card and paying for your clothes). That way, you always have the information handy when you need it. When you are at the store and you see that incredible sweater, you can check your list and see whether you really need it, or should you be absolutely positively certain that you have to have it, you can to consult your wish/want/need list to see what is the best color to buy.

Wish/Want/Need List

Wish/Want/Need Items	Color	Size

18

Scents-ible Advice: What You Should Know About Perfumes

*Perfume is the unseen but
unforgettable and ultimate fashion accessory.
It heralds a woman's arrival and
prolongs her departure.*

—GABRIELLE "COCO" CHANEL

Fragrance: A Mood in a Bottle

Movie actress and perfume designer Elizabeth Taylor is quoted as saying, "Fabulous fragrances, like fabulous jewels, add mystique and confidence to every woman." My sentiments exactly! So when my ex-boyfriend Derek went away to visit with family back East the summer before our senior year in high school, I was confident that his getting a periodic whiff of my perfume would keep his thoughts of me alive and well.

Since I couldn't be with him in person (although believe me, I really wanted to!), I had to settle for writing him every day. To make absolutely sure Derek didn't forget me, I scented all the letters I mailed to him with my favorite per-fume. It was the perfume I wore on all our dates. I had no doubt that when Derek smelled the scented pages, he remembered me—and our times together. I was certain it made him long to be with me again, which, of course, was just the effect I was going for! Though Derek didn't put cologne on his letters to me (that's not something too many guys do, although I really don't know why), I remember his favorite cologne as well: Polo. To this day, if I smell a guy wearing Polo, I dreamily think of the ways I felt for Derek.

Use Sense with Scents

There's no doubt that fragrance wields a power over us. I'd like to think the perfume I spritzed on my letters to Derek that summer is one of the reasons why he called me every time he received one of my letters.

Even the research proves the power of perfume. Olfactory research (the study of the effect of "smells" on people) shows that certain scents can make people feel relaxed, excited, sensual, happy and even productive. Psychologists, for example, have found that peppermint and lily of the valley are stimulants and when these scents are sprayed in the rooms where students are taking tests, the students are more alert and score higher than when they are not used! Because it has been discovered that certain aromas make a difference in the level of employee productivity, many Japanese firms mist certain fragrances into the air within their offices. For example, when a jasmine fragrance is used, employees have a 21 percent drop in error rate in the products they produce; with lavender, a 33 percent drop; and an astounding 54 percent fewer errors with lemon wafting through the air! Other scents are valued for their relaxing properties. Researchers at New York's Sloan-Kettering Cancer Institute have found that the scent of vanilla can relax patients. In short, scents have capabilities to change our moods and influence our actions. I know Derek's mood was certainly influenced each time he got my perfumed pages!

The Rule: The Earlier the Hour, the Lighter the Scent

Because scent has such a powerful influence, you have to be careful how you use it. Perfume can make others enjoy being around you . . . or run for cover when they can smell you five minutes before you arrive! I think the absolute worst is people who feel that wearing perfume (or cologne or after-shave) is a substitute for taking a bath! Use scent to enhance, not to disguise. The rule is, the earlier the hour, the lighter the scent.

A lot of people have the mistaken idea that "if a little bit is good, more is great." Colleen, a classmate of mine, doused herself with her favorite musk-scented perfume every day. I could hardly handle being in the same room with her. Sitting next to Colleen for even twenty minutes would give me a headache. When Colleen left the room, her perfume remained behind for what seemed like hours. It was never hard to find where Colleen was or had been in school—you just followed your nose! Now, it wasn't that the perfume smelled bad or anything; it was actually very nice. The problem was overkill because Colleen was using way too much. (A word of warning: Perfume can stain your clothing, so don't douse your wardrobe.)

A girlfriend of mine told me that her mother always said, "No one should be able to smell your perfume unless he's close enough to kiss you!" I don't know whether I'd go that far, but I agree that perfume should be a very personal thing. If the students on the other side of the classroom start putting clothespins on their noses, or pass out when you're around, you know you've doused yourself too much!

Pulse Points: Where to Wear Perfume

How do you know how much to put on? International perfume expert Jan Moran (and author of *Fabulous Fragrances,* a wonderful book that tells you everything you ever wanted to know about all perfumes created to date) says that one dab of perfume should be applied on the pulse points. A pulse point is a part of your body where your pulse is strong. Each time your heart beats, or the pulse throbs, a little bit of perfume is sent into the air. Good places are behind each ear, and on each wrist and at the bend in elbows and knees and in the hollow of your throat. Some people like to spray a little mist all over their necks. Again, if you're in close quarters, like the classroom or a movie theater, go easy.

It's also fun to put scent on a place where that special someone is sure to notice. My friend Kiley has really beautiful hair, which her boyfriend loves to touch. Naturally, she spritzes a little perfume on top of her hair (when he leans over her, he smells it). And Selena, another friend of mine, likes to smell her own perfume and so she puts a dab on her hands. When she is not wearing perfume she uses scented hand lotion made from the same perfume.

Why You Can't Smell Your Own Perfume

Keep in mind that it's hard to smell yourself. This is because of *sensory adaptation,* meaning you get used to a smell when you are around it a lot. You know how when something really has an odor to it, it bothers you for only a few seconds, then you don't notice it so much anymore—like the smell of a certain food, or even your pets? I have two kitties and am very meticulous about keeping their litter box clean. But the other day, when a friend was visiting, she walked into my house and remarked, "Jennifer, you need to clean out the kitty box!" I can no longer smell my kitties—but others can!

The same adaptation happens with perfume. When you've been wearing the perfume for a while (sometimes for only a minute or two), you don't smell it anymore. This past month my mother and I

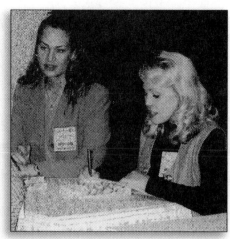

Mom and I at an Orlando booksigning for Taste Berries for Teens.

were in New Orleans at the American Library Association doing a book signing. All of a sudden the air was filled with a glorious scent of perfume. My mother looked up and said, "Oh, someone smells simply wonderful!" At her saying this, the woman first in line looked around to see if she could detect the scent my mom was smelling. "I don't smell anything," she said. My mother and I looked at each other and naturally had to laugh because the woman looking around was the woman wearing the glorious-smelling perfume. But, she was so used to wearing it that she could no longer smell it! "What are *you* wearing?" my mother asked the woman. "Giorgio," the woman replied. "Oh, it's one of my favorites!" my mom told her. "I love the floral scents!" "Me, too," the woman said. "I've been wearing it for I don't how many years. Whenever my husband doesn't know what else to get me for a gift, he gives me perfume. I must have six unopened bottles, so I'll be wearing it for a long time!" Hmmm. I think the woman brings up a good point. Maybe we need to teach the guys a little about our other favorite perfumes. If the guys you know are like the guys I know, they don't know too much about the different scents.

The problem with getting used to the perfume is that you put it on and think that the fragrance isn't strong enough—so you dab on some more. Suggestion:

If you are used to your perfume and are considering adding more, ask your friends. The scent may already be strong enough. A simple, "Do you like the smell of my perfume," or, "Can you smell the perfume I'm wearing?" will get you the information you need to know if you are using too much.

How to Be Scent-sational

Have you noticed that the exact same perfume or cologne can smell one way on one person and either subtly or entirely different on another person? This is because each of us has her own individual body chemistry, which can interact differently with the ingredients in any given perfume. My mother has a favorite scent, and to me, the smell of her perfume is simply glorious. Every now and then when we are traveling together I'll ask her if I can use her perfume. She always says yes—and always, no one compliments me on how I smell when I wear it. But they do compliment me on my own perfume.

Perhaps a cologne you admire on a friend smells awful on you. Or your favorite perfume seems different in winter than in summer, different still when you're happy or upset, ill or feeling at your very best. Those differences aren't imaginary—weather, body chemistry and even mood can affect fragrance. Your mood and the temperature outside (how warm or cold it is) all affect how a fragrance smells on you. You may even notice a change in the way your favorite fragrances smell on you if you've changed your diet, if you're taking a new medication, if you're under more stress than usual or having your period.

Here are some other interesting facts about perfume.

- People with a higher proportion of body fat retain scent longer.
- People with oily or darker skin retain a scent longer than do those with dry or paler skin.

- Fragrance evaporates more quickly during exercise, or if your skin is dry, or if you are on a low-fat diet, or if you live in a cold climate.
- Your body emits more of the perfume you are wearing when you perspire or spend time in warm temperatures.
- The sun spoils the oils in perfume and changes the way it smells. If you carry perfume in your purse and carry your purse with you when you spend time in the sun, then the heat can alter your fragrance. Instead, leave your perfume at home, or if you do take it to school, put it in your locker.
- Experts say it is a good idea to store expensive perfumes in your refrigerator. At home, store your fragrance bottles away from direct sunlight and extreme heat. You might set it in a drawer or beneath the sink in your bathroom. If you put it in the refrigerator, be sure to place it in a plastic bag or else other foods in the refrigerator will smell like your perfume! No matter how much you like the scent of your cologne, I'm sure you'd rather have your pizza smell like a pizza rather than your pulse points!

Coordinate Your Perfume with the Colors of the Season

Did you know that King Louis XV loved the smell of fragrances so much that he demanded that his court wear a different perfume for every day of the week? Fragrance experts say there is no such thing as one perfume that fits all people, or each person all year long. You already know that you use scents to match your mood—or your boyfriend—but there's another commonsense consideration in deciding what perfume to wear: What season is it?

Experts recommend you select a heady floral or an oriental fragrance in the winter; in the summer (or if you live year-round in a warm climate) select a lighter floral or citrus scent. The goal is to chose a soft, light cologne or an eau de toilette. On a crisp fall day, try a *chypres* (a warm sweet smell of oakmoss or a woody scent) because it best matches the mood and "feel" of the season. When spring returns after a long winter, go with a "green" perfume—these smell clean and fresh, and match everyone's mood for a season that Robin Williams so aptly epitomized when he said, "Springtime is nature's way of saying 'Let's boogie!'"

In the information above, did you find yourself thinking that wearing a perfume shouldn't be all that complicated, and wondering who could possibly get it all straight anyway? It may sound complicated, but it's not. Once you understand even the basics about the six different categories of scents, your idea about perfume will forever change. The next section explains the essence of understanding the six different styles of scents. Don't forget to teach your boyfriend this information. If he's a guy who likes to give his girl perfume for her birthday, chances are he'll give you a perfume (his choice) in the "category" of scents that works well with you. And here's another way to use this information: When someone (like Mom, Dad or your grandparents) asks you what you want for a birthday, add perfume to your list—especially those that you love but can't afford to buy for yourself just yet!

Top Notes, Heart Notes, Base Notes: Styles of Scent

There are a few basic categories of scents. Each of these is as different from the next one as one primary color is from another. Each category is based on the main theme of the scent, for example, *floral* or *spicy*. When you get an idea which division of scent works best on you, you can narrow your search down to colognes in that division and avoid wasting money on scents that wind up unused in a drawer, only to be tossed out a year later.

- Floral fragrances are the largest category of scents. Many are made up of single flower scents although more are being created with multigarden flowers such as rose, gardenia, carnation, jasmine, honeysuckle and hyacinth. Floral scents are fresh, soft and sensual and make you smell like what else—a flower! Popular fragrances include Joy, Giorgio, Chloe, DKNY, L'Air du Temps, White Diamonds, Champs-Elysees, Amarige, Escada, Calyx and 273. Florals have a springtime and cool, summer-day smell—one I grew up around; my mother is a Spring.

- Oriental fragrances are heavier, richer and spicier scents. They are made up of exotic resins such as incense, musk and spices. These scents are often considered ideal for cool weather and evening wear. Classic examples of perfumes with this kind of scent are Shalimar, Opium, Angel, Guess? and Obsession. Winter girls love Oriental fragrances because they smell so divine on them.

- *Chypres* (pronounced "sheep-ra") is French for cyprus. *Chypres* scents have a warm and sweet smell are often described as woody-mossy. They're created from earthy substances such as oakmoss and sandlewood. Classic *chypres* scents are Versace, Paloma Picasso, Y, Ysatis and V'E Versace. I love to wear Versace in the fall to beach parties. That mossy smell works perfectly with a mohair sweater worn around a crackling fire. I'm an Autumn girl, and my favorite perfume of all is Cartier—another *chypres* scent.

- Green scents are those that bring to mind the fragrance of a freshly mowed lawn or a walk in a forest—pine, juniper, sage. It's a real summer scent. If you are a Summer girl, probably you find yourself adoring scents in this category. Classic examples of green scents include Di Borghese, Aliage, Pheromone and Tommy Hilfiger's Freedom for Her.

- Citrus scents are the fresh, sharp, clean fragrances that provoke thoughts of citrus fruits, such as tangerine, lemon, orange, grapefruit and lime. While they are often thought to be mostly men's fragrances, classic examples of their use in women's perfumes can be found in Eau de Hermes, Diorella, Eau de Patou and Eau de Guerlain.

- *Fougere* (meaning fern in French), pronounced "foozh-air," is an interpretation of fresh green ferns, with a hint of lavender, citrus and oakmoss. *Fougere* ingredients are most often used in men's fragrances, but it is also a scent worn by women. Many of the "his and her" fragrances contain the ingredients commonly used in *fougere* scents. This is a relatively new division, so to date there are not many perfumes in this category, though Jicky is a popular one with teens.

Each of these scents are further broken down into classifications, shown below. I won't elaborate on each one here, but should you be interested in knowing more, you can check out the suggested reading section for this chapter at the back of the book. You can also ask a salesclerk at the perfume counter for a profile of fragrances by scent type. Knowing all about perfumes is their business, and it's been my experience that they sincerely want to help you find a perfume you'll enjoy.

Subclassifications of Perfumes

Florals: green, fruity, fresh, aldehyde, amber and oriental
Oriental: amber, spice
Chypres: fruity, floral—animalistic, floral, fresh and green
Citrus: none other
Fougere: none other

What perfume belongs where is determined according to its ingredients. To help manufacturers come up with a new scent, and to help buyers know what is in the perfume, each fragrance is further divided into "Notes" according to dominant ingredients. The most potent ingredients, the ones setting the tone for the fragrance, are called top notes. The secondary ingredient(s) are called heart notes, and the lesser ones are called base notes. Let's take Bijan for an example:

Top Note: ylang-ylang, narcissus, orange blossom
Heart Note: Persian jasmine, Bulgarian rose, lily of the valley
Base Note: Moroccan oakmoss, sandalwood, patchouli

When you factor this information in, then what you can decide is not just if you are a floral, but rather a floral-oriental. If you are, then scents like Bijan are exactly the scent you want.

Whew! Never knew there was so much to just smelling good, did you?! If you find all this fascinating, you aren't alone. When I tell teens about it in workshops, they are amazed at how they *already know* this information on a working level; knowing *why* affirms what they have already experienced.

The knowledge can serve you well in other ways. I once bought a bottle of perfume simply because it smelled incredibly wonderful on the clerk at the fragrance bar in a department store. That's not such a good idea. After making the purchase, I spritzed it on and then continued shopping. Within half an hour I had a real headache—and got one every time I wore that perfume!

Nor is it a good idea to buy a perfume because a sexy, glamorous ad announces the latest and hottest trend and promises that it's the surest way to get your dream date to ask you to the latest hot concert tour when it comes to your town. Fashion is fun, but let your nose be the authority on what scent is right for you regardless of the trend. Select what is best for you and most appropriate for the occasion.

So how should you buy a perfume? The following section can help you make the right choice.

The Nose Knows: The Three Levels of a Perfume's Fragrance

Just because you like a first whiff at the fragrance bar in the store doesn't mean that you'll appreciate the scent when you take it home. That's because scent changes over time. Fragrance in fact has three distinct levels.

The first level of a perfume can last from thirty seconds to three minutes. While a fragrance is usually purchased based on the impression this level gives, this isn't the scent that you'll be wearing in the end.

After the first level of scent wears off, you enter level two. This middle-level fragrance lasts up to ten minutes. If you put on perfume a few minutes before your date arrives, you are at the second level of the scent by the time you go to greet him and climb into his car.

Level three of a fragrance is called the "dry down." This scent is what you smell for several hours after you apply the scent. Obviously, this is the main level of the scent, the level that lasts the longest. Therefore, it is wise to wear a scent twenty minutes or more before you buy it. Since the aroma will be going through these different levels, you'll need this time to know whether or not you really like the way it smells on you over time. Perfume expert Jan Moran says it's not a good idea to try on more than three fragrances at a time in the store when you are trying to find one you like. Why? Because your nose gets overwhelmed and you really won't be able to decipher the difference between the scents.

So as you can see, when it comes to selecting a cologne or perfume, impulse shopping is not a great idea. Try a fragrance, go away and do some shopping for an hour, then come back and buy it if you still like the way it smells.

As time passes, your body chemistry also changes as you change your activities. For example, in the morning you may be sitting in your biology class dreaming about the cute boy in front of you, but by the afternoon you are in gym class doing just five more crunches trying to top your personal record. A scent that worked well when you were sitting still in the morning may not work so well when you are huffing and puffing in the afternoon. Therefore, it's a good idea to take home samples when they are available. That way, you can have more than one trial run for smelling the scent, wearing it in different settings.

This also gives you a chance to see if the scent is right for you in other ways. For instance, does wearing it for a long time give you a headache? Remember how I mentioned earlier that my friend Colleen's musk gave me a headache when I was around her? Even the nicest cologne, your favorite one that you love wearing, can be too much after a few hours. When you try a perfume, keep reapplying it every few hours for a day and keep track of whether you have any reaction. Do you feel slightly dizzy or nauseated? Are you getting a little pink rash where you applied the perfume? Each of us has a unique body chemistry. While you may be able to wear most colognes, there's always a chance that one simply doesn't work with your body.

The Aroma of Your Home: Scents in Your House

Have you ever heard of something called *aromatherapy?* You know that aroma means scent. Therapy is healing or curing or treating. Aromatherapy, therefore, is making someone feel better using scent. Think about how often this happens to you. You walk in the house, tired after a hard day of school. But wait! Is that freshly baked chocolate-chip cookies you smell? That great aroma makes you start grinning as you dash to the cookie jar, and your mood is better even before you take the first bite. Maybe you enter a room that has just been cleaned with a pine cleaner, and you enjoy the "outdoors" smell of a fresh home. Do you (or your parents, friends or boyfriend) use a scented refresher in the car? I do. I use one that smells like strawberries, because I love the smell of them. My boyfriend uses a car deodorizer that gives off the same smell as a brand-new car.

Aromatherapy is nothing new. For hundreds of years people have used scents and essential oils taken from herbs and flowers to heal headaches and depression, to relieve stress and to improve the memory. The use of scent has been shown to create greater physical and emotional health. If you're having a rough time, going through a lot of stress and need a pick-me-up, why not try some aromatherapy yourself? Here are some ways you can use scents to make yourself happier and maybe even healthier.

- Use potpourri. Potpourri is a mixture of dried flowers and spices. It often comes in a bowl and can be found in all sorts of scents from heavy and musky to light and floral. I keep a dish of light potpourri right by my bed. When I swish the flowers around, the scent renews itself. I find the smell helps me to relax and sleep better. Here's a tip. As the roses in your garden (or from that special someone) begin to fade, pick off the petals and put then in a bowl (or nylon) and spray them with perfume. Most girls love this personal way to keep the petals from a special time, a special someone. My mother does this for me, and every time I smell them, I think of her and all the ways she loves me. I also keep a separate bowl for the flowers I receive from guys. The only problem is, when I break up with a guy I don't like the reminder and so I toss the potpourri—and hence precious dabs of perfume!
- Burn scented candles. Candles are very inexpensive (much less expensive, in general, than perfumes or colognes) so you can use a lot of them, especially while soaking in a bubble bath! **Caution!** Don't fall asleep with the

lighted candle burning. You don't want to end up burning your house down.

- Scent your drawers and closets. You can find sachets (little scented pillows of cloth, usually no larger than a few square inches) in all sorts of scents. You can even make your own by dribbling a couple of drops of your favorite cologne on a piece of cloth. If your perfume bottle is empty, don't throw it away—open it up and put it in your drawer. There is enough scent left to make your clothes smell great. You can also rub a little perfume oil directly on the wood inside your drawer.

- Use fragrance on your pillows and sheets. It's so great to go to bed at night with sheets and pillows that smell like your favorite perfume. Just think of the pleasant dreams you'll have!

Buying Scents with Sense

How much should you pay for great smells? It depends on your budget. But you may need to shop around. You can find some wonderful bargains on good perfumes in discount stores, chain stores and drugstores. There are also a number of "designer" fragrances that are far less expensive than real perfumes. These are generally an imitation or scented oil. Designer fragrances can be good for regular school days and activities, but as a rule, their fragrance doesn't last as long as cologne or true perfume.

The more fragrance oils used in a formula the longer the fragrance will last—and the higher the retail price will be. *Parfum* (or perfume, they mean the same thing), is the most intense form of fragrance.

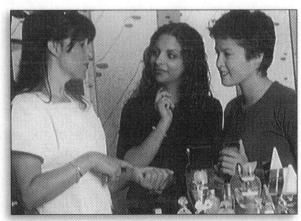
Inquire about perfumes before you buy.

This is followed by *eau de parfum, eau de toilette* and *eau de cologne*. These last two terms, eau de toilette and cologne, are virtually interchangeable.

Consider trying eau de toilette, especially if you haven't worn a particular scent you are thinking about buying. Even though it is not as intense as the stronger version of it will be, the eau de toilette is a good way to test it before you invest a lot of money, and until you're sure you like the way it smells on you. The difference between perfume and eau de toilette is that a perfume is made with natural and expensive oils, which, being heavier, hold the scent of the perfume much longer than an eau de toilette, which is made with less expensive ingredients, such as alcohol and other substances. An eau de toilette is therefore much cheaper ounce for ounce, but once you have it on, it will wear off in a fraction of the time that perfume would.

Breaking News: You Heard It Here First!

With just a bit of research and shopping around, you'll be sure to find just the right fragrance for the best money. Felicia McCree, a manager at one of the many Body Shop stores, says teens should keep on the lookout for some great *new* fragrances about to hit the market. "The *Street Scent* fragrance collection is developed especially for the trend-conscious teenage girl," she says.

Street Scent has four fragrances: Cosmic Candy, Citrus Rush, Virtual Cherry and Forbidden Fruit. All are available in a fragrance, body spray, shower gel, lip gloss and nail color! Wow! They sound delicious! Just remember, you heard it here first!

Smelling wonderful and knowing it, smelling wonderful and getting great compliments for it, can do everything from making you feel good about yourself to setting the mood of a dinner out with your friends. Try it for yourself!

In the next chapter, you'll learn how to dress up even more—like fixing your face and hair, and some other ways to work magic with cosmetics.

UNIT FOUR
Skin Care, Hair and Makeup Magic

*If you get simple beauty and nought
else, you get about the best
thing God invents.*

—ROBERT BROWNING

Inventory: Magic for Sale— Makeup Magic, That Is!

Remember when you were just a little girl and being able to put on your mother's lipstick was such a glamorous thing to you? Even back then, you knew how important such details were when it came to being beautiful. Just as you imagined it would be when you were a little girl, one of fun things about being a grown-up girl is that you've entered the magical land of brilliantly designed little bottles that contain every potion possible. How fun! It's just one of the many benefits of being a girl. So, if it were as simple as waving a magic wand, which of the items below would be "gotta haves" for you?

- ❑ Brown hair
- ❑ Black hair
- ❑ Blonde hair
- ❑ Red hair
- ❑ Curly hair
- ❑ Straight hair
- ❑ Longer hair
- ❑ Shorter hair
- ❑ Thick, shiny, healthy hair
- ❑ A flawless complexion
- ❑ Perfectly straight teeth
- ❑ Whiter teeth
- ❑ A great smile
- ❑ A year-round tan
- ❑ Never having to wear makeup
- ❑ Soft, smooth, beautiful hands
- ❑ Tons of makeup in every shade
- ❑ Long, thick, curly eyelashes
- ❑ Perfectly shaped lips
- ❑ Beautiful eyes
- ❑ Expressive eyes
- ❑ To be one of those girls who knows how to apply makeup "just perfectly"
- ❑ Soft, smooth skin on my entire body
- ❑ Nails that never break or chip

❑ A makeup makeover with the world's most famous makeup artist

❑ Beautifully shaped eyebrows

❑ A new hairstyle and makeover by Hollywood's leading stylist

❑ A facial any time I want one

❑ A manicure and pedicure any time I need one

When it came right down to it, did it seem like so many of these "details" were important enough to warrant a purchase? You want thick, shiny hair *and* a flawless complexion! A great smile is a real asset, but you also want beautiful eyes! Alas! Even Cinderella had a few restrictions imposed up on her—like her coach turning back into a pumpkin if she wasn't home by midnight! (That would probably be a bit much to explain to a new date!) Your limitation? Absolutely none!

In this unit, you'll learn how to use your beauty wand to work magic to enhance your each and every feature even more! After all, there's a Cinderella in each of us.

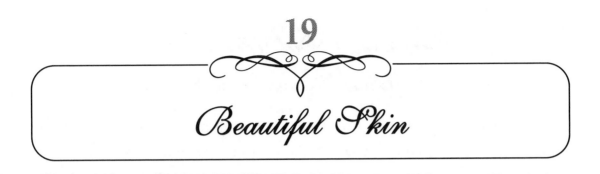

19

Beautiful Skin

*Beauty is truth, and
truth, beauty.*

—JOHN KEATS

Face Value:
A Beautiful Complexion

You are standing with friends outside of a movie theater, waiting your turn in line to go in. A girl about your own age comes walking toward you to join a friend of hers who is already in line. What is the first thing you notice about the girl approaching? The style of the outfit she is wearing? Her shoes? Her smile? The color of her hair? Her jewelry? How physically fit she is? Her demeanor?

Probably it's a combination of these things, but chances are, after an initial overall glance, you focus on her face. You notice the shape of her nose and mouth and maybe the color of her eyes, but even more so than the appeal of her facial features, you specifically notice her complexion. Incredible, isn't it, that the quality of what is "skin deep" can speak so loudly as a first impression. Yet it often does.

Heirlooms: Did You Inherit Your Complexion?

Everyone compliments my mother on her beautiful complexion. She always replies by saying, "Thank you. I inherited it from my mother, and she inherited hers from her mother." There's no question that heredity can have a lot to do with the nature and appearance of your skin. A good friend of mine, Evan (who is sixteen), has a very serious case of acne—just like his father had when he was a teen. "Runs in the family," he says whenever someone reminds him of the remains of the lotion he applies to his face to heal his acne. I've met Evan's father. Judging from the deep scars on his father's face (the result of a

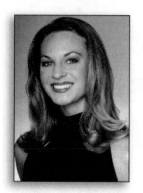

serious case of acne he had in adolescence), it's easy to see where Evan inherited his skin condition.

But beautiful skin is more than good or back luck. Good genes are not enough to ensure that your skin will stay healthy just because you've been born with a great potential for smooth skin. And just as Mom or Dad had troubled skin doesn't mean you have to be stuck with complexion problems.

You need to take care of your skin. It begins by proper care and grooming.

Skin 101: What You Should Know About Your Skin

Understanding your skin can be valuable information. Here's a quick overview on how and why your skin is what it is, and does what it does. Your facial skin is several layers deep. The outermost layer of skin is called the *epidermis.* The epidermis is made up of two layers, a "dead-cell" and a "live-cell" layer.

As gross as it sounds, the "dead-cell" layer is what you see when you look at someone. It has an important role to fulfill: Because it comes into direct contract with the external environment, this layer is our first line of defense in doing things like making the skin waterproof. It also shields the delicate "infant" cells at work growing beneath it. This layer contains cells called *keratinocytes* which vary in thickness depending on their location. For example, the skin around the eye area is only about as thick as a sheet of fine paper, while that covering our heels may be as thick as a piece of leather. You are constantly shedding this layer of dead cells. These cells fall off when you shower or rub your skin with your hands or a washcloth. They slough off as you dry your face with a towel, and most especially when you exfoliate your skin (discussed later in this chapter). Pores, narrow channels that lead into a *sweat gland* or a *sebaceous gland,* are found in this layer.

The next layer of your epidermis is made up of living cells. These living cells divide over and over again, constantly producing new skin cells. As they do, the older cells are pushed to the surface—where they begin their function as a dead cell! This layer of living cells also contains *melanocytes* or pigment cells. These generate melanin, which is responsible for the color of the skin. The more melanocytes we are born with, the darker our skin, hair and eye color will be. In addition to being genetic, melanocytes can be triggered by sunlight. When you go in the sun, melanin darkens, and presto! You have a tan.

The next layer, the *dermis,* is a thick and very tough elastic layer. It contains the blood vessels bringing nutrients to the skin and carrying waste products away. Your body's nerves endings are also found in this layer, as are sweat and oil glands and hair roots. The primary purpose of a sweat gland is to aid the body in perspiring—one of the ways the body attempts to cool you down. The job of the busy little sebaceous gland is to produce oil that keeps the skin soft and flexible. It is this same gland that produces the oil to moisturize your hair and keep it healthy and shiny! This health of this layer is immensely important to the vitality—beauty—of the outer layer of skin. The effects of inadequate nutrition, exercise, rest and relaxation, as well as the effects of smoking, take their biggest toll here.

Next comes the *subcutaneous* layer, which is composed primarily of fat. Like the other layers, it's important and vital to our health and beauty. Among its many roles, this layer acts as a cushion to absorb shock (such as if you were to fall down or get hit), thereby protecting the inner organs from being traumatized. And, of course, it is this fat that helps give our face and body form, and, generally, lies at the heart of a comment such as, "She's too thin."

These important layers are charged with the same things to do through-out our lives. However, during adolescence, the oil glands in the skin begin to produce more oils than they normally do, which is the biggest reason adolescence is a time when acne and other skin disorders are most common. And this is why being a teenager means that you must care for your skin and do those things that keep it at its best. Dead skin cells, grime, makeup and perspiration can block a pore from breathing. When this happens, a plug forms that blocks a pore and thus causes pimples—blackheads and whiteheads.

When you think about all the skin does, it's really quite miraculous. You can best help it be beautiful by understanding the job it has to do, and by doing your part to keep it healthy.

The drawing below shows the skin's basic makeup and its duties:

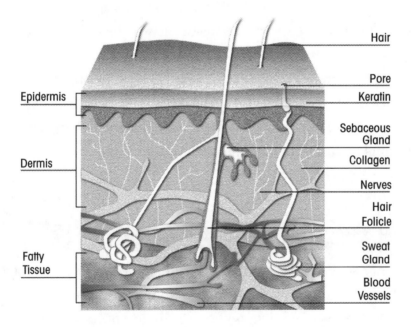

Getting the Glow: The Essentials of a Beautiful Complexion

The expression that "beauty begins on the inside" is especially true when it comes to your complexion. Drinking plenty of water, eating a healthy diet, getting enough rest, and exercising regularly are essential to the health and appearance of your skin. This may sound like the "same old, same old" advice you heard from your parents as a youngster, but as a teenager when you really need to look great all the time, nothing could be more important than to put into practice these commonsense but vital basics. As every skin-care expert will tell you, "If you take care of the inside, it will take care of you." Some things, it seems, never change.

Later on in this chapter, I'll give you more detailed information on how to properly care for your skin so that you can look your best, especially through the hormonal ups and downs of adolescence. For now, here are the basic beauty treatments to have healthy and great-looking skin—sans makeup!

Beauty Treatment # 1: Water It!

Drinking plenty of water is one of the best things you can do to have a nice complexion. Water is an essential part of the human body (nearly 80-plus percent in fact). Like air, we can't live without it. In addition to helping the body distribute nutrients, water also helps your system flush out toxins and impurities. Drink at least eight glasses of water a day. After doing this for even three to four days, you will notice a big difference in the appearance of your skin. It will look healthier; at the very least, it will look well rested.

Teens often ask me if soft drinks, teas and cappuccino can be counted in their eight glasses of daily liquids. Sorry, but nothing is a substitute for the pure water your body needs daily. In fact, drinking fluids that contain caffeine, like sodas and coffee, for example, actually dehydrates your body. This is why doctors recommend that for every eight ounces of these types of beverages you consume, you need to drink an additional twenty-four ounces of water.

Here's a tip: If you find that drinking water is "boring," as most teens tell me it is, and your taste buds need a little encouragement to down the eight glasses of water your body needs on a daily basis, try adding a flavor [as suggested in chapter 8] to give a little pizzazz to the water.

Beauty Treatment # 2: Feed It!

Your diet and nutrition play a very important role not only in keeping your skin healthy but in giving it a clean and smooth and "glowing" appearance as well. Your skin is a living, breathing organ (it's the body's *largest* organ); it needs nourishment. In addition to adequate nutrients, it needs essential vitamins, minerals, amino acids and enzymes to function properly.

Feed your body foods that keep it healthy. A diet that is deficient in certain vitamins, minerals and nutrients can upset body chemistry. If your diet consists mainly of sweets or greasy foods, for example, your skin is going to react to these things. Just as not getting enough sleep shows up in tired-looking skin, especially under the eye area, the quality of nutrients you are supplying to your body shows up in the condition of your skin. Likewise, when your diet properly nourishes your cells, your skin is more likely to radiate health. For more information on the foods to best fuel your body, refer to the chapters on diet and nutrition in this book.

Making sure your skin is nourished properly also means no smoking. Smoking causes your blood vessels to constrict and this reduces blood flow throughout your body. Your skin has a big job to do in keeping you healthy—and alive. Among its many functions, it keeps you properly hydrated by regulating salt and water through the sweat glands. It's your body's thermostat, cooling you down and warming you up when needed. It flushes impurities from your system through the blood vessels, oil glands, sweat glands and pores. It filters out the sun's UV rays so you don't burn up.

We may think of our skin as an aesthetically appealing wrapper for our body, protecting all those internal organs so they can do their jobs, but in reality, the skin is the body's largest and busiest organ. Always looking out for us, when a skin cell begins to tire it's sloughed off, growing a new one to take its place. But as self-sufficient as it is, your skin depends on you to do your part so it can do its important work. Your skin depends on blood flow to bring the nourishment it needs. Smoking starves your body of nutrients, water and oxygen it needs to do its many task. And, smoking dehydrates your body, leaving your skin dry and pasty looking, and speeding up facial wrinkles. Be kind to your skin: don't smoke.

Beauty Treatment # 3: Exercise It!

Better overall health is one benefit of exercising. Vibrant glowing skin is another. Just as our bodies need adequate amounts of the proper nutrients to sustain good health, our cells depend on oxygen to function and do their work. Physical activity is the key. Physical activity increases our circulation, carrying oxygen-rich blood to the cells so they function efficiently.

Exercise really does improve the appearance of your skin, especially your complexion. My skin is always more radiant on those days after a workout than when I go several days or even a week without working out. The equation is a simple one. More oxygen circulating throughout the body keeps the cells in better condition. Good circulation speeds up the turnover of your skin cells; this helps give you fresh, healthy cells at the surface of your skin. Healthy cells means better health, a vitality that shows up in the form of beautiful skin.

Beauty Treatment # 4: Rest It!

Is sleeping one of your favorite things to do? Most teens would say yes to that question! Good news: Getting your beauty sleep is one of the skin's most important beauty treatments. How well rested you are shows in your skin. Sleep deprivation shows up in your complexion, especially in the fragile skin around your eyes, giving you dark circles and puffiness, and making you look tired and drawn.

So how much sleep do you need? Health experts say that teens need eight to ten hours of sleep each night to support the intense stage of growth and development. Added to your body's natural need for sleep, you need even more rest to keep up with your busy schedule and all the stress and strains of being a teenager. For more on the importance of sleep to your overall health and for ways to rest and relax the body, check out the chapter on rest and relaxation in this book.

Beauty Treatment # 5: Keep It Clean!

Keeping your skin clean is essential to having beautiful skin. Pollutants and grime in the air, makeup, as well as your body's own production of natural oils, need to be cleansed away, especially at the end of the day. When sweat, oil or dead skin is not washed away, pores become clogged and can cause skin irritations, such as rashes and acne. Clogged pores can stretch your skin, making pores larger and resulting in a ruddy appearance. Cleanse your skin.

Five Steps to Kissable Skin

1. Why and How to Cleanse Your Face

Washing your face is an important part of your skin care. *How* you wash it is important to your skin's health and beauty as well, and can spell the difference between having skin that is dry and looks tired, even dirty, and having skin that looks radiant and healthy—in a word, beautiful. You know this and head to the store to get yourself a good cleanser. You approach the aisle of beauty products only to discover that it's not that simple. There are literally dozens upon dozens of products claiming to help you have beautiful and kissable skin. If working your way through the maze of all the different brand names isn't perplexing enough, then the decision of which one is best is for your skin will be: soaps, scrubs, cleansing creams, astringents, exfoliants. How's a girl to decide which is right and best for her skin-care needs?

For starters, keep your eye on the goal. Your skin produces its own natural oils as a way to keep itself healthy. Your goal is to cleanse your skin, without removing these essential oils. Secondly, select a product that is right for your skin type; is it normal, dry, oily, or a combination of these? Keep in mind that your skin needs change over time, depending on the climate, your lifestyle and even according to your hormonal changes. And remember that expensive isn't necessarily better. Read the label; look for a cleanser that says it does what you're trying to achieve: reduce oil, add moisture, cleanse only, and so on.

There are many cleansers to chose from. Here's a quick rundown:

- **Bar soap** (also known as *milled* soap because of the way it is produced). It's made from tallow and vegetable fats. To jazz up this basic and simple soap, lathering agents and fragrances are generally added. If you have oily, normal, or moderately dry skin, this will probably suit your needs. A word of caution however: the skin around the eye area is thin and fragile so don't "scrub" this area.

- **Superfatted soaps.** As their name suggests, these soap products contain lanolin and cocoa butter that give them a high fat content. They are gentle to the skin so if you have sensitive or relatively dry skin, a product containing superfats may be right for you.

- **Transparent soaps.** These are much the same as superfatted soaps except that they also contain ingredients like glycerin and alcohol that makes them translucent. Because of their high fat content, if you have oily, sensitive skin, this type of soap product should work for you. However, if your skin is very dry, don't use these products; the alcohol content can dry your skin even more.

- **Deodorant soaps.** These products blend soap with antiseptics that control bacteria and hence reduce body odor. These products are great for bath and shower, but because they are drying to the skin, never use them on your face. While it might be easier to just use whatever bar of soap is in the shower while you are showering, these products are too harsh and can also irritate the skin, making it more prone to sunburn and wind chafing. They can even cause a rash. If you dry out your skin too much, it will flake—and that's no fun. Whenever I have a peeling nose from too much sun, or a flaking forehead because I've been overzealous in applying an astringent, I'm self-conscious. I also know I've been "mean" to my skin.

- **Medicated soaps.** These products boast of containing ingredients specifically aimed at combating problems like acne and eczema. Unless your dermatologist or doctor has suggested you use one, you might as well save your money. You aren't going to leave soap on your face or body; once you wash away the soap, gone too is the medicating action.

- **Detergent soaps.** Because these are made from petroleum products and fatty acids, they tend to be less irritating than many other categories of soaps. They are oil-based, so if you have normal, dry or sensitive skin, these should work well for you.

- **Organic soaps.** These feature natural ingredients like plant extracts, vitamins and minerals. Save your money. Applying these ingredients to the outside of your skin offers no benefits to your skin whatsoever. Because they are packaged in such an appealing way, they look nice on your counter top though! If you are buying them for use, read beyond the rah-rah of "added" ingredients, such as plant extracts, checking to see what else they offer in the way of cleansing.

- **Exfoliating soaps.** These contain grains of pumice or crushed volcanic rock or cornmeal (among other things) that chafe the skin so as to remove dead cells. Though popular products, the dermatologists I consulted agreed that such products are too abrasive and too drying to be used *daily,* especially since our bodies are in a continual state of sloughing off dead cells on their own. In addition, we slough them off ourselves as we wash with a washcloth and dry with a towel.

- **Scrubs.** Scrubs rely on abrasive particles that also remove dead cells, but also offer emollients to moisturize the skin. There are tons of these products on the market. If you decide to use one, read the label carefully. If it is alcohol-based, it can dry your skin. If it is oil-based or water-based, it won't offer much in the way of cleansing your skin.

- **Masks.** Facial masks cleanse the skin by removing oil, grime and dead cells. Though masks are designed to do different things, from adding moisture to soothing tired skin, essentially they are drying and most effective if your skin type is very oily. There are two types of masks, those that wash off and those that peel off. Wash-off masks are usually made up of clay-based ingredients, while peel-offs contain chemicals that dry and then are gently peeled off your face. Both tend to sap moisture from the skin as they work their magic of lifting impurities from your face, which is why it is recommended they not be used more than once a week, if that.

- **Astringents.** These products use ingredients such as alcohol or witch hazel to "tighten" and "refresh" your skin. Boric acid, zinc, menthol and eucalyptus are often added to give your skin a tingling sensation. It's mostly hocus-pocus. Astringents offer no cleansing and no long-term "tightening," and can cause irritation and allergic reactions for those with dry or sensitive skin. Astringents are most useful for giving your skin the appearance of smaller pores, but only for a few hours. Be aware of the trade-offs.

- **Cleansing creams.** These products are more of a makeup remover than a cleanser. There are oil-based products (like Ponds, which my grandma uses)—typically wiped off your face with a tissue. Water-based products (also called foams, gels, gelees) are typically rinsed off. With either one, you should wash your face after using it (most especially if you have oily skin) because they leave a film on your skin that you will want to remove so it doesn't clog your pores.

So there you have it. Different products (I've profiled only the major ones!), many brands to chose from. Again, read the label; the pretty packaging should not be your consideration, nor should you buy the same product just because your best girlfriend uses it. Understand what you are trying to accomplish, and then once you get the product home, use it as directed. If it says to leave on for a minute and you leave it on for fifteen, there may be consequences, such as drying your skin more than you wish, or causing a rash.

It's a good idea to wash your hands before touching your face. Your hands touch everything: Don't transfer the germs on your hands to your face.

The best way to cleanse your face is to wash your hands first and then splash lukewarm water (or pat it) on your face. Using your hands, gently apply soap or cleanser to your face, working up a lather. Leave on for about thirty seconds (or as directed) and then rinse your face thoroughly with cool water. Gently pat your skin dry with a clean washcloth (this saves on laundry). If at all possible, avoid using your soiled bath towel on your face.

Now you're ready to apply a toner.

2. Why and How to Use a Toner

Makeup, perspiration and the grime in the air form a film on your face and slow (even stop) your body's natural oil from working its way out of the pore as it normally would. Your pores can also get clogged if you don't remove your makeup at bedtime. Your pores need to breathe. Clogged pores can cause your pores to enlarge over time. (Even using overly warm water enlarges your pores.) As you recall from the material above, astringents are generally over rated and not considered to have long-lasting results. They do, however, provide a short-term solution in reducing the appearance of large pores. Because of their ingredients, toners tend to be drying to the skin, so if you decide to use one, don't overdo.

What should you look for when buying a toner? There are a good number of brands on the market. Brand name isn't at all important. Look for a toner that doesn't contain witch-hazel, alcohol or fragrance because these ingredients are drying and can irritate your skin. This is especially true if you have thin, fair or sensitive skin, or if you spend considerable time in the sun or in dry environments, like the classroom.

Do not apply toner to your entire face. If your skin is both oily and dry, use a cottonball to apply toner to your chin, nose and forehead only. Known as the "T-zone," these are the areas with the most oil glands.

Don't rinse your toner off. It's okay to apply makeup over it.

3. Why and How to Use a Moisturizer

Do *teens* need to use a moisturizer to replace lost moisture and avoid dry skin? There are two schools of thought here—no, and yes. Professionals are really divided on what they think is best for teens. Some dermatologists are adamantly opposed, while some say it's an okay idea but an unnecessary one. Still others agree with other skin care specialists such as facialists and say it is an absolute must.

First the argument against teens using a moisturizer: The skin derives its moisture from our sebaceous glands. Arguably, most teens have fairly active sebaceous glands and so their skin is adequately protected from being too dry; consequently, teens have little reason to add moisturizer.

The argument for adding moisturizer is this: Our skin going about its daily duty in caring for itself may not be sufficient to combat the wear and tear of our lifestyle in today's high-tech time. Air-conditioning, overhead lighting, more frequent exposure to hot and cold temperatures, a greater emphasis on fitness (and playing sports and spending time in chlorinated pools) and hence dehy-dration from perspiring—all take an extra toll on the body's natural production of oils. Therefore it's smart to use a moisturizer (and most especially if you are using a medication to combat acne). So what should you do? My advice is to know your skin and make a deci-sion based on what you think is right. For example, when I was in high school, I con-stantly played sports, was always outdoors, and my skin was on the dry side. I needed to add moisture. I'm going to provide you with the scoop on moisturizers so you can decide for

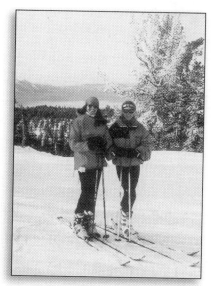

It's a smart idea to use a moisturizer with sunscreen when you're outdoors.

yourself. And, of course, if you are unsure if using a moisturizer is best for you, ask a dermatologist or skin-care specialist.

Most moisturizers are advertised as "daytime use" or "nighttime use." The difference is that a daytime moisturizer usually has a sunscreen in it and is not as creamy (so makeup will go on over it). For daytime use, you want a moisturizer with sunscreen to protect against the damaging effects of the sun to your skin. Even if you are working on a great tan, you definitely want to use a moisturizer (as well as makeup) with sunscreen protection. Most makeup brands have only SPF-5UV (ultraviolet) protection, so the moisturizer you select should have at least SPF-10 of sunscreen protection. If you don't wear makeup, select a moisturizer with a minimum SPF-15 protection—which is the minimum guideline recommended by skin-care experts. Dermatologists and other skin-care specialists agree that the very best sunscreen contain these three ingredients: avobenzone, parsol 1789 and zinc oxide (more about this later).

Moisturizer versus Emollient

Sometimes you'll see a moisturizer advertised as an emollient. The difference between a moisturizer and an emollient is this:

- Moisturizers add moisture to your skin. Some contain ingredients to heal skin conditions, such as a rash or sunburn.
- Emollients are made of oils and silicones that seal in moisture and make your skin softer.

Some moisturizers include emollients. You'll pay a little more for these, but in my opinion, they're worth it. Sealing in moisture is really preferable to simply having soft skin, especially since emollients will soften your skin, too.

How often should you use a moisturizer? It really depends on your skin. If you are trying to combat oily skin, it only stands to reason you won't want to overdo it. And besides, if you slather moisturizer on, you can actually clog your pores, creating blemishes. If your skin is very dry, you will want to use moisturizer after thoroughly cleansing your skin. If you are like me, and you spend considerable time in dry environments—like the outdoors, or even in dry indoor air, like the classroom—you'll need to moisturize even more often. But as a rule, you'll gauge your need to moisturize your skin according to when it needs it. For example, if you are on the swim team and spend time in chlorinated pools, or if you've just returned from three days on the ski slopes, chances are your skin is drier than normal. And, right around the time of your menstrual cycle, your skin is extra oily, so you may not need to moisturize during this time. Be attentive to the needs of your skin.

Helpful Hints for Using Moisturizer

- Don't overdo. If you layer on too much moisturizer, you will clog your pores, making them larger, and even causing blemishes to appear.
- Unless your skin is extremely dry, apply moisturizer only to the areas that are drier than the rest of your face, like around your eyes (or around your nose area if you've had a cold and have been blowing your nose so frequently that it's resulted in overly dry skin).
- When moisturizer is applied over damp skin, it creates a thin film that allows the skin to absorb the moisture into the skin, and that's a plus!

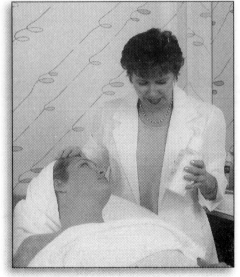

Skin-care expert Karina Pawlukiewicz and me

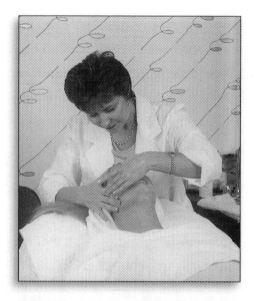

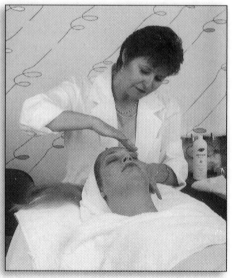

- Always apply your moisturizer (as well as makeup) to your face in gentle, upward and outward strokes. This is a good habit and will serve you well all your life. Gravity, age and normal wear and tear are what cause the skin to lose its elasticity and hence eventually sag, so begin now in your teen years to treat your skin gently. Why add to the problem of your skin's eventually losing its elasticity? Believe me, you will always be grateful that you practiced prevention.

- Do not use a petroleum jelly or baby oil to moisturize your face. Petroleum jelly and baby oil (as well as moisturizers that have mineral oils) clog the pores, causing skin disorders such as whiteheads, blackheads or deep underground pimples. When excess oil combines with the outer layer of the skin, the pores get clogged, causing you to break out.

4. Why and How to Shed Your Skin: Exfoliation

Trees shed their leaves in the autumn. Many animals shed their coats from season to season. Likewise, our skin also sheds, sloughing off the old cells as it makes way for the new cells. Skin experts say we shed more than a million cells every day!

Skin that is shedding is dry and looks dull. New skin is fresh and clean looking. Makeup, perspiration and daily grime from the environment can mean our skin can use some help "turning over a new leaf." It's called exfoliation. Exfoliating is a step beyond cleansing the skin of makeup and daily grime. It's a deliberate attempt to "go for the glow!" Be careful though. Over-washing your face will remove too much of the oil your skin naturally needs to be healthy. And if you scrub your skin too briskly, you will overstimulate your skin.

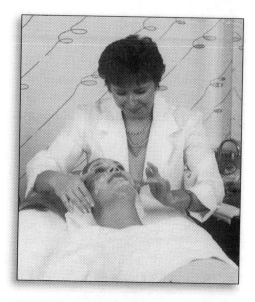

I use a "Buff-puff" (a small sponge especially designed to gently scrub the face) every other day in my regime of cleansing my face. The important thing is to massage ever so lightly and in circular motions. Again, facial skin is fragile.

If you can afford it, I highly recommend that you get a facial every six to eight weeks from a skin-care expert. While the price of this service will vary from salon to salon depending upon the length of the procedure (a thirty-minute facial versus a ninety-minute facial) and the types of products used, as an average, a facial will cost between $50 and $75 (be sure to ask

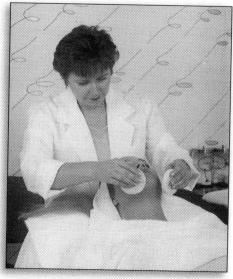

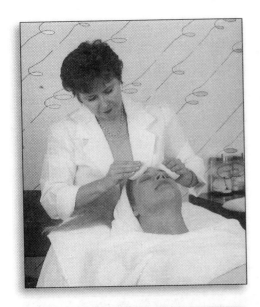

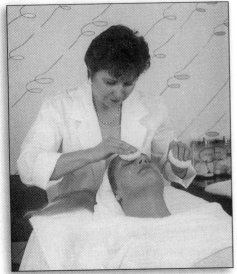

before you schedule so you know what to expect). Once you find a facialist, it's also a good idea to return to her regularly for the care and treatment of your skin. One reason for this is that she will know your skin type and know how your skin responds to different products, so, if your skin changes from, say, over oily to over dry, she'll know how to best help you restore your skin. As an example, for a number of years I have been going to Karina Pawlukiewicz at Karina's European Skin Care. I like her services for several reasons: She is a real pro, her skin-care training is extensive, she is wonderfully personable, and she always best advises me on how to keep my skin healthy and in good condition—in spite of my lifestyle. So if I'm just off the ski slopes and my skin is dry and crying from the windburn and high-altitude sunburn, Karina knows exactly how to soothe it and get it glowing again. If I've been ten days abroad touring and conducting workshops, usually the change of time zones and spending hours upon hours in airplanes mean I'm exhausted and my skin is suffering from dehydration and sleep deprivation. Once I'm home, Karina is among my first calls, because my skin needs rejuvenation as much as I do.

Get in the habit of treating yourself to a facial now, and your skin will be forever grateful. I had my first facial when I was in the ninth grade. It was a birthday gift from my mother. After that, I always looked at my allowance differently, knowing that a portion of it was going to be held in reserve for a facial whenever I could make my money stretch that far. It was money well spent. Throughout my high school years, Karina rescued my skin from break outs (from stress or hormonal imbalance); restored it from the drying effects of having spent hours playing sports in the sun; as well as buffed and shined it to a high gloss for a special occasion like class pictures or prom night.

Care for your skin properly and it will reward you by looking healthy and radiant.

5. Why and How to Detoxify Your Skin: Facial Masks

When I was in high school, a group of us girlfriends would often have a slumber party, an overnight get-together where we would analyze the latest gossip at school, discuss who was going out with whom (or wanting to), and compare notes on the latest in fashion trends and makeup tips; you know, hang out. We would do this while in pajamas as we were listening to music, especially the latest hits—and wearing our "faces" (facial masks). Of course, having all dipped into the contents of the same jar, we all wore the same look. We even took turns as to who was to bring "the goop" (facial mask).

This meant that Jeanne, a girl with a very oily complexion, wore the same facial mask as Marianne, a girl who was on the all-state swim team and swam two hours each and every morning—in addition to swimming twice a week in competitive swim meets and sometimes even on the weekends. Spending so much time in chlorinated pools was very drying to Marianne's face. If one of us had brought a mask designed to dry one's face, this was good news for Jeanne but not so good for Marianne. And if the "goop of the day" was for adding moisture, this would be good news for Marianne but not for Jeanne.

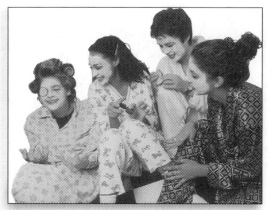

"Purely girlie" necessities!

The rest of us, with skin somewhere in between that of Jeanne and Marianne, fared little better than either of the two of them. We had no clue that masks were manufactured to do a specific thing—like dry out or add moisture. To us, a mask was a rite of passage—something the big girls did—especially those as cool as we were! Because this was our ritual, and because we really didn't know any better, we simply took pleasure in putting on "our faces" (cucumbers on our eyes, included!).

Needless to say, this is not the way to use a facial mask. Because of our different skin types and depending on our particular skin-care needs, we would have been better served if we had each purchased our own facial masks based on the needs of our skin, and simply brought them along to our slumber parties and each worn our own. And of course, there are those who would argue that a mask is "purely girlie" and not all that beneficial to keeping teen skin healthy and glowing. How useful a particular mask is to cleansing your skin depends on the type of mask you are using and how you use it. On the fun side of things, no girl would disagree that friends who come together and apply their "faces" experience a very special bonding. With our "faces in place," we are all equal in every way!

Facial masks are designed for any number of skin-care reasons. There are masks to *detoxify* your skin, which means to draw the toxins and impurities out; masks to *add moisture*

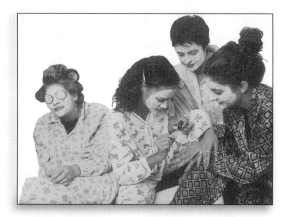

With "faces" in place!

to your skin; masks *to help rid your skin* of excess oils; masks to *soothe* irritated and sunburned skin. There are masks to *deep clean* your skin, and masks to cool your skin, to *pamper* it. Not all masks designed to do exactly the same thing are equal. Each can use any number of different formulas and ingredients. For these reasons, don't just buy one because it's handy, or on sale. Read the label carefully: What is it designed to do? Are you allergic to any of the typical ingredients found in masks? I found out the hard way. Several months ago, I used a mask that contained iodine and developed a mild rash. It wasn't until I used the mask a second time and had the same reaction that I discovered I was allergic to the ingredient in the potion. Always test the formula by placing some of it on your underarms, because that area has the same type of skin as the area under your eyes. Wait twenty-four hours before you determine whether or not it causes any reaction before actually using it on your face.

If you'd like to try a mask but are unsure what to purchase, you might talk to your mother. Does she use a mask? Does she suggest one for you? You might also ask your family doctor or a dermatologist (a medical doctor trained in the care and treatment of skin), especially if you are considering purchasing a facial mask to combat a skin condition such as acne. (Because there are different degrees of acne, always consult a dermatologist to determine what is the best way for you to care for your skin before you resort to remedies on your own.) Another way to determine if a certain kind of mask is recommended for your skin type is to ask a skin-care specialist, such as a facialist at a respected beauty salon or a consultant at the makeup counter in a reputable department store.

Beauty Treatment # 6: Treat Problem Skin

A pimple in the middle of your face on the day of the big dance ranks right down there with getting dumped by your best friend or seeing the boy you like holding hands with someone else. Zits are the pits. Unfortunately, breaking out is a very common problem for teens because in adolescence, the oil glands in the skin begin to produce more oil than they normally do. The result is skin bumps, zits, acne.

Acne is a condition in which the oil glands become blocked, infected and swollen, resulting in whiteheads, blackheads, pus-heads (pustules) or cysts. What's the difference? To understand why these unwelcome guests intrude upon us, you need to understand that it's all about fluids from the oil glands needing to escape through the pores. If fluid cannot escape the opening of the oil pores (because it is clogged with dead skin cells, perspiration, bacteria or sebum—the cells' natural lubricant—or if the pore is simply closed), a *white-head* results. Because the skin is not inflamed, usually these are not painful. A *blackhead* develops in much the same way, only taking its name because of its darkish coloring (derived from your own skin pigmentation) as it makes its way from the sebaceous gland to the oil pore. The blackhead, too, is usually not painful because it isn't inflamed, which is not the case for a *pus-head* or *pustule*. The pustule (the medical term sounds so much better!), on the other hand, is inflamed, therefore it hurts.

Basically, a zit comes about because the cell is trying to discharge its natural oils and by-products and they can't get out. When this happens, the cell fills up with the accumulated oils and bacterial waste products, and because these cannot escape, it swells and eventually, erupts—or tries to. Sometimes these skin conditions get better with self-care and other times they will need to be treated by a dermatologist or skin-care specialist.

A dermatologist is a skin specialist, a medical professional with special training in all areas pertaining to the skin, and can help you with the most effective way to treat your problem skin. This is especially important in cases when bacteria has infected or blocked the pores, causing cysts or boils.

The A, B, C and D Grades of Acne

There are different degrees of acne, and dermatologists use a grading system to distinguish between mild, moderate and severe cases.

Grade A is a mild outbreak of whiteheads and blackheads. Typically these are not inflamed and the best way to treat them is through proper cleansing. You can also buy an over-the-counter cleansing product specifically designed for acne-prone skin. Usually these will contain one (or a combination) of these ingredients: benzoyl peroxide, alpha-hydroxy or salicyclic acid.

Grade B (very typical for teens) is a moderate case of whiteheads and blackheads as well as pustules or pus-heads—inflamed zits. Depending on how your skin reacts to self-treatment, you may wish to consult a skin-care specialist.

Grade C is an outbreak of whiteheads, blackheads and deep-seated pastules on the face, neck, chest and shoulders. You will definitely want to seek medical attention to treat this skin condition.

Grade D, just like the D in school, requires your utmost attention—and the care of a dermatologist. These deeply embedded cysts are very painful and can cause permanent scaring if left untreated.

In caring for problem skin here are some other things to remember:

- **Keep your skin clean.** The best first line of defense against blemishes is clean skin. If your skin is extra oily, wash it with a mild facial soap two or three times a day. In addition to cleansing your skin, you might ask a pharmacist at your local drugstore for help in finding the best over-the-counter skin medications. He or she may recommend products that contain agents that will kill bacteria, as well as treat mild cases of acne.

- **Don't overwash!** While it's important to keep your skin clean, if you wash it too much you can strip it of natural sebum (oil) and it may respond by overproducing oil, which leads to blackheads and pimples.
- **Treat the "T-Zone."** If your skin is exceptionally oily, use an astringent over your "T-zone" area during the day, as well as at bedtime. Remember to cleanse your face first.
- **Don't squeeze.** Skin-care specialists recommend that you not squeeze blackheads, so don't. But if you do, be extremely gentle. If you press too hard you can break skin tissue, and cause an infection, even scarring. Always make certain that the skin is clean. Wrap a tissue around your fingers (this prevents germs passing from your hands to the open wounds) before lightly applying pressure. Afterwards apply a light pat of an astringent (you can buy this at any drugstore). An astringent is used to kill bacteria and germs, and to gently dry the area in order to help it heal.
- **Take good care of your overall health.** Make it a lifestyle to eat healthy foods, and get adequate exercise and rest. Learn positive ways to manage your stress. Strive to be happy. And remember, if you feel your breaking out is not because of your diet and cleansing routine, and that your complexion is taking a turn for the worse, ask your parents if you can see a dermatologist. At the very least, go see your school nurse. As always, talk to your mom and dad about your concerns for keeping your skin healthy.

Your Skin—And Its Monthly Moods

Many teens find that their skin is especially susceptible to breaking out about a week before their menstrual cycles. This is due to heightened hormonal activity and can generally be controlled by drinking plenty of water to flush out your system. (Don't worry that drinking a lot of water during a menstrual cycle will make you retain more water. The truth is, it'll help flush out the water you are retaining.) Though I've come across some dermatologists who say there is little correlation between the foods we eat and breaking out, as a rule, most concur that it is wise to minimize greasy and fatty foods, as well as candy and chocolates during this acne-vulnerable time. Moderate exercise will also help your circulation do its job, as well as reduce your PMS moods swings.

Beautiful Skin—All over Your Body

The skin on your face isn't the only skin you want to be healthy and beautiful. The skin on the rest of your body needs TLC, too.

(You Are Never Too Young to) Fake a Bake

Unfortunately, just as the sun gives our skin a nice glow, it can also cause great damage, making our skin to become leathery, wrinkled and discolored. And, overexposure to the sun's ultraviolet (UV) rays can cause skin cancer. Tanning lamps also produce this damaging ultraviolet radiation. While much of the advertising coming from the tanning salons suggests there is no risk to damaging your skin, skin doctors tell me tanning beds are positively devastating to your skin in the long run. If you are trying to get an update on the safety of tanning salons in your area, check with a local dermatologist. He or she can best advice you what is best for your long-term skin health.

In general, the darker the skin, the less sensitive it is to ultraviolet radiation. So the fairer you are, the more committed you'll want to be to faithfully using a good sunscreen. But no matter if you are fair-skinned, dark-skinned or somewhere in between, dermatologists recommend using a sunscreen of at least SPF-15 UV protection. In many cases, you will need a sunblock to block solar radiation.

What's the difference? A sunscreen *filters* out the rays, while a sunblock stops all rays from penetrating your skin. When looking for one, read the label. You'll see a Sun Protection Factor (SPF) rating. This is a standard rating used to help you decide what level of protection you are seeking in order to keep from being burned by the rays of the sun. It's a system that allows you to judge for yourself what protection you need. For example, SPF-15 is a common number, meaning that if you were in the sun without any protection at all, wearing SPF-15 should allow you to stay in the sun fifteen times longer without burning. Common sense—and the strength of the sun, and the length of time you are in it—then, dictates which is the best one to wear. If you are going for a late-afternoon bike ride with your friends, an SPF-6 sunscreen *may* be adequate. If you are going to spend the afternoon water-skiing, you may very well want to wear an SPF-30 sunscreen, or better yet, wear a sunblock.

Here are some other important reminders in protecting your skin (and hair) from the harmful UV rays of the sun:

- **Avoid taking a blast of radiation.** The sun gives off its strongest radiation at twelve noon, which means that anytime between ten and two you need to protect yourself from the damaging effects of UV exposure.
- **Don't let the clouds rain on your (life) parade.** Don't be fooled by cloud cover; while they offer us a little protection, they don't filter out all the harmful UV rays.
- **Shop with the sun in mind.** If you are extremely fair—like a redheaded friend of mine—it's wise to wear more UV-resistant clothing. Many sporting-goods-stores carry clothes that are especially designed to protect delicate skin. Woven fabrics like cotton, polyester and rayon block out UV rays better than do open weaves such as gauze, linen and cotton knits. White or light-colored clothes also do a better job of screening out rays than do darker colored clothes. And, get in the habit of wearing hats,

preferably wide-brimmed hats made out of tightly woven straw or other fabrics. These offer more protection than do loosely woven fabrics. Caps are always a cute look, but unfortunately, they don't always offer protection for the fragile skin on the your ears, throat, and neck, and even some parts of your face.

- **Protect your eyes.** Invest in a great pair of sunglasses, ones that offer your eyes the protection they need from the sun. If you have dark eyes, you may need less filtering that those with light-colored or sensitive eyes. Expensive isn't necessarily better. Again, read the label. Protect your eyes.

- **Keep your lips kissable!** Don't forget to protect the delicate skin on your lips from the UV rays. Look for a lip balm (or lipstick) designed for protection from the sun.

Be good to your skin. Keep in mind that your skin doesn't have to be decades old before it succumbs to skin cancers. Protect it and it will stay healthier longer. You can have a great tan without paying the price of the harmful effects of the sun.

How to Look Like a Bahama Mama—Without Leaving Home

You don't have to bake in the sun to get a great-looking tan. Whether you're hoping to achieve the look that prompts your friends to ask if you got your color sitting in the stands at your sister's afternoon soccer game, or to wonder if you went to the beach with someone special, you can get the ultimate sunless tan—from a tube. There are some really great (sunless) formulas on the market, ones that don't leave your hands stained and won't wear off in those telltale streaks when you shower or perspire.

Usually those lotions designed to be used on the face contain different ingredients from those used on the body. Many teens like some of Lancôme's

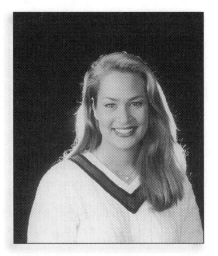

Diligently care for your skin.

formulas because they won't cause you to break out (though this feature is sure to be in most of the products trying to win over teens). Whatever brand you use, once you've determined the shade you want for below the neck, complement the shade of your body with a self-tanner or liquid bronzer for your face, or you can skip the self-tanner in favor of a sweep of bronzing powder. I like the brand Aveda Bronzer Minus Sun for a "sun-kissed" look, but there are a lot of them on the market.

For below the neck, I like Neutrogena Sunless Tanning Spray; Estée Lauder Go Bronze or Yves Saint Laurent Long-Lasting Radiant Primer in Brown Copper for a medium tan. For formulas that get others to rave about how dark you are, you might try Bain de Soleil Deep Dark Streak Guard or Clinique Self-Tanning in Dark. On your face, enhance with bronzy foundations, like Bobbi Brown Bronzing Stick in Dark or Ultima II See-Thru Shimmer blush stick. Again, these are my favorites and I only provide the brand names so you can see how popular "tube tanning" is compared to the harsh rays of the sun. The goal is to take care of your skin.

Taking care of your skin shows you care about you and your good health. A word of caution: Should you notice any spots on your skin, discoloration, unusual freckles, moles, or warts, have them checked by your doctor or a dermatologist. At the very least, show them to your parents so they can help you decide if seeing a doctor is the right thing to do. Chances are they harmless, but prevention is the best policy—and a sign that you are serious in protecting your health and well-being.

Alligator Skin? Shedding with a Loofah Scrub

Do you sometimes feel that your skin belongs to an alligator? Just as you can stimulate the shedding of old skin and replacement of new on your face, you can also exfoliate the skin on your entire body by gently scrubbing with a loofah sponge or a shower mitt while you bathe or shower. A loofah sponge is a natural sea sponge that is dried out. A shower mitt is usually made out of a ropelike fiber, though sometimes they are made out of plastic in the shape of short bristles. I personally like the hand mitt because it's easier to use. I've tried the plastic bristles, but they're too scratchy for my skin. You can find a loofah sponge or shower mitt at almost any drugstore. They are inexpensive, usually under $10, and last five to six months. The plastic one will last forever!

Unlike your routine of using a soft towel to pat your face dry, following your shower or bath, dry off with a coarse towel. Briskly rub your skin. Doing so is good for circulation and helps slough off dry skin as well. Get in the habit of doing a body scrub every other time you shower. It will keep your skin looking a little pink at first, because circulation is increased. And, as a reminder, extra rubbing to the backs of your legs and buttocks is still the most effective way to minimize cellulite.

If you do this for several weeks, you'll notice that your skin has a healthy glow. This is because you are stimulating the skin to shed the dry skin and to replace it with new skin. Then, apply a moisturizing lotion or cream after you dry off.

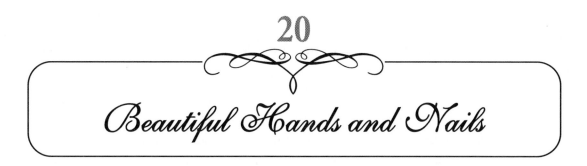

Beautiful Hands and Nails

*The sky will bow to your
beauty if you do.*

—Rumi Jelaluddin

Tara Shipley

Tara Shipley, a senior-high friend of mine, is a very busy girl. Along with being a catcher on her school's softball team, Tara volunteers to coach a Little League team for her community center twice a week. Her school team meets every other day for practice, and competes against other schools every other week (sometimes on the weekend). Tara also works part-time at the local nursery where, in addition to her duties at the cash register, she helps customers box up and then carry their plants, soil and gardening supplies to their cars. Even with all these jobs that require her to use her hands, Tara has beautiful hands and nails, as I noticed once again the other day as she and I were looking through CDs at the store together.

Hands: How to Keep Yours Soft and Pretty

I know how hard it is to keep your hands and nails looking nice when you are as active as Tara. I love the outdoors and go horse riding as often as I can. Part of caring for my horse is the feeding and constant grooming—brushing, combing, washing and cleaning his hoofs. All these activities are very drying to my skin and take a toll on my nails, as well. Yet I need to have smooth skin and nice-looking nails in the work I do, which entails a great deal of time in front of an audience as I conduct workshops—to say nothing of the scrutiny my nails get as I do book signings—or when my hands are being kissed by a special guy!

Hands are high visibility: You raise your hand in class; you wave to people. You use your hands to punctuate your conversations and express yourself, you reach out to touch others and even to shake hands with someone to whom you've just been introduced. For better or for worse, the condition your hands are in make an impression on others. Whether your hands are playing sports, taking a quiz, relaxing at the pool or being held by a special someone, the condition of your hands and nails reveals to others how much you tend to yourself.

Beautiful hands are well-groomed hands. Here's how you can keep yours looking their best:

- **Always keeps your hands clean.** From holding hands to shaking hands, from using our hands to guide us down stairwells to guiding our stroke in putting on our makeup, we touch and handle everything. Wash your hands with a soap that contains a *mild* disinfectant (this is to kill bacteria). You will find disinfectant hand soaps sold in most drug stores and grocery stores.
- **Dry your hands thoroughly.** This helps them from chapping and from drying out as well. Use a clean paper towel, washcloth or hand towel

(soiled, moist towels have bacteria you really don't want back on your clean hands) to dry your hands.

- **Moisturize your hands after you wash them.** Keep a bottle of hand lotion beside the sink in the kitchen and one by the sink in your bath area. Get in the habit of dabbing on moisturizer immediately after each time you wash and dry your hands.

- **Stimulate circulation.** Whether applying moisturizer or watching TV, get in the habit of massaging your hands, particularly your cuticles. This gets the circulation going and is good for the skin. I keep a small tube of hand lotion in my purse for convenience so I can massage my hands when I have a little extra time, such as when I'm waiting for an appointment.

- **Use a moisturizer at bedtime.** If your hands are particularly dry, apply extra moisturizer and then wear lightweight gloves (or socks) on your hands overnight. You should be able to find gloves specifically made for this use in beauty-supply stores and in the beauty-supply section of most drugstores as well.

- **Get in the habit of wearing latex gloves,** if your family responsibilities (dishes, clean-up duty), part-time job or hobbies are such that your hands are frequently in water. This can prevent your skin from dehydrating (losing precious moisture necessary to their being soft and supple); shield your skin and nails from the harsh effects of detergents, disinfectants or chemical agents being used in the water; protect your nails from breaking; and if you wear nail polish, it can help prevent it from chipping.

- **Learn how to manicure your nails properly,** so that not only does the appearance of your nails add appeal to your hands, but so that you care for your nails in a way that promotes their being healthy (more on this in the next section).

Letting Your Fingers Do the Talking: Caring for Your Nails

Did you ever wonder why we have fingernails and toenails in the first place? Why don't the tops of our fingers and toes simply resemble the bottom sides? The answer is simple: Our nails have a very important role in keeping us healthy and in protecting our well-being.

The portion we trim, file and polish is the *nail plate*. It is primarily made up of hardened layers of keratin (and other things, like sulfur), and its primary purpose is to protect the vast numbers of intricate nerve endings as well as the multitudes of blood vessels at work below, carrying nutrients and oxygen to the tips of our fragile fingers and toes. The portion of the nail plate we see is made of nonliving cells. The nail plate extends up under our skin. This portion is called the *nail matrix* and is made up of living cells. We do see a little portion of the nail matrix, however; it's the little white half-moon-shaped portion and because of its shape is called the *lunula*—a Latin word meaning half-moon. The *cuticle* is the dividing line between these two, and serves to prevent infection and bacteria from invading the nail matrix. The cuticle is so important to protecting the overall health of the nail that while we often trim it, we shouldn't. Most dermatologists will tell you that gently pushing the cuticle up and under is the best practice in caring for your nails. In most cases, this is also sufficient for giving a nice appearance to the nail.

How to Do a Great Manicure

Manicuring our nails is not only how we keep them pretty, but healthy as well. Give yourself a manicure every eight to ten days or as often as you need to. If you can afford to have them done professionally, do so every couple of weeks—in addition to your own self-care maintenance in between. Most salons charge in the range of $9 to $15. If you can't afford a manicure, and don't like to do your own nails, have a girlfriend do them—and then you can do one for her. A manicure is not only good for your nails, it makes for a great "girl session" with a best friend.

Here are some tips on how to give yourself a manicure:

1. **Start with the right tools.** The basics: Fingernail clippers; cuticle keeper (get the kind with a rounded and slightly sharp edge to push cuticles without damaging them); nail file; three-way buffer (get the kind that has extra-fine surfaces for getting nails smooth); emery board; orange sticks (these often come in a package of six or twelve and double as a cuticle pusher and polish correctors); base coat (to help polish adhere and to fill in any irregular surface of the nails); nail polish in several colors (including clear); quick-dry polish formula; polish-preserving top-coat; nail-polish remover (acetone free if you can find it); cotton swabs to remove old polish; isopropyl rubbing alcohol (to sterilize your tools before and after each use).

   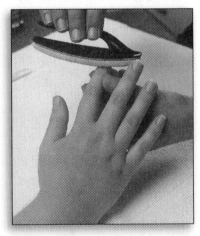

2. **Remove old polish.** Always use a moisturizing remover, preferably one that is acetone free, because this abrasive chemical is extremely drying and potentially damaging to the nails. Using a cotton ball dipped in remover, gently wipe from the base of the nail outward. *Gently* is the operative word here: If you press hard, you will bruise your nails. (If you've ever done this, you know

   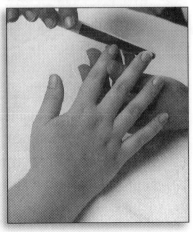

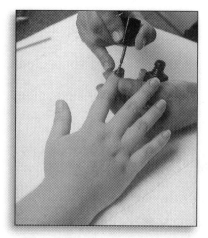

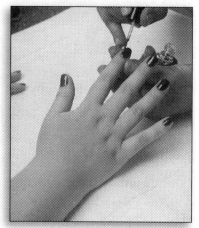

from experience that it hurts.) If at all possible, avoid getting remover on your fingers. You really don't want your body to absorb this harsh chemical—and it is harsh, no matter what it says on the label. Manufacturers have yet to come up with anything strong enough to melt or dissolve nail polish without using a potent chemical, so until they do, exercise caution and use sparingly. (The moment a gentler and better-smelling nail-polish remover product is developed, buy it immediately!)

3. **File your nails with an emery board.** File in one direction, not in a back and forth motion. This will prevent your nail from chipping and splitting, which will weaken the tips of your nails, causing them to chip and break easily. Though the shape of your nails is a matter of personal preference, a square-shaped nail is less susceptible to breaking, splitting and chipping. When filing, be gentle so as not to damage your nails: The thinner your nail, the finer the emery board should be. Unless your nails are very long, it's better for the nail to be filed than it is to be cut with a clipper. The reason is that this is less traumatic for the nail plate.

4. **Attend to your cuticles.** Use cuticle softener (such as moisturizer or cuticle oil), applying it to the edges of your nails and massaging it in gently. Using an orange stick (not cuticle clippers), gently push the cuticle away from view. Don't cut "in" to your cuticle because that will cause it to bleed. Clip any hang nails, but do this gently, being conservative in how much skin you remove. (If you have been trimming your cuticles or getting a

professional manicure and the manicurist has been trimming them, ask her to instead use an orange stick.) While cutting the cuticle is standard practice in many salons (though not all), it is not good for the health of your nails.

5. **Use a cotton ball dipped in an astringent** (like lemon juice, though alcohol works, too) **to remove any excess oil**. This will make your polish go on smoothly without bubbling.

6. **Apply a base coat.** This will make your polish stick better and will fill in any irregularities in your nail. Stroke from the base of the nail to the tip. Let this base coat dry before applying nail color.

7. **Use a one-coat polish, brushing it on in smooth, even strokes.** Look for a polish that contains both a color and a top coat. It's a great time-saver, and it works better than using two separate products (though you should apply two coats if you are using standard nail polish).

8. **Correct mistakes.** If you aren't as steady-handed as you'd hoped, you can correct a mistake by dipping a cotton swab in polish remover and carefully trace the skin around the nail, rolling the swab as you go so the cotton stays clean.

9. **Add a seal coat.** If you are using an all-in-one polish, one that is both a polish and top coat, then add a seal coat. This helps protect the finish and adds a high-gloss look. Stroke from the base of the nail to the tip of the nail, wrapping down under the nail. This will add a protective sealer and help prevent chips.

It's a wise idea to go without polish for two to three days before painting your nails once again. Giving your nails a break from polish not only gives your nail plate a chance to breathe and repair itself, it also gives it a break from the staining caused by adding color to your nails. (Because nails are porous, dark nail polish stains more than do pale or clear colors.) If your natural nails looks faded or yellowish in color, one reason may be because the color of your nail polish has stained the nail plate (check to be sure you have a good base coat—which should prevent yellowing—and are applying it correctly). Another reason may be because you have an infection (yeast infections are most common from nail polish). Should you notice that the yellowed nail appears crusty or that the nail is splitting and peeling, you need to see a doctor as soon as possible.

Imitation Limitations

I was at a restaurant last week having lunch with Siena Tarkington, a good friend of mine. As we were paying for our lunches, I watched with amazement as the cashier used the eraser end of a pencil to literally tap our tab into the cash register. The woman had on nearly two-inch-long fake nails—I kid you not! They looked more like a bear's claw or an eagle's talons than a human's fingernails! To make matters worse, they were painted in a deep, dark purple, and each one studded with a different-colored rhinestone. As elaborately decorative as I'm sure her manicure was meant to be, it wasn't pretty. My next thought was that the plastic extensions covering her natural nails got in the way of her doing her job. It also struck me how lucky I was that this employee was at the cash register—and had not been in the kitchen preparing my food! Her nails not only looked like a disadvantage in her work, they also looked unsanitary. Keeping your hands and nails well groomed and cared for is a part of staying healthy! And looking your personal best.

What You Should Know About Fake Nails

Personally, I don't recommend that you get fake nails for a couple of reasons. First of all, the teen years are a good time to be really active and involved in any number of activities, and artificial nails can be a hindrance to getting involved and doing these things. Take sports for example: The physical work-out is a great way to keep in shape and burn off tension, as well as to help level off the oftentimes runaway emotions caused by all the hormonal ups and downs. Team sports especially can win you friends; being together, striving together, competing together builds respect and admiration for each other. The benefits are simply too good to miss out on.

The teen years are also an important time to be involved in all sorts of hob-bies. After all, this is a time when you are in an active search to find your inter-ests and talents and trying to find an interest big enough to pursue as a job, work or even as a career. Again, these years are so important—too important to miss out on—and most especially because you are having to be protective of your fake nails. When I was in high school, the girls who wore artificial nails always seemed to shy away from certain activities for fear of breaking or tearing a nail. A good friend of mine wore her artificial nails so long that she couldn't even use the camera to snap a photo. I thought of her nails as a limitation to the fun the rest of us were having. The girls who went out for sports or really enmeshed in other activities, on the other hand, couldn't be bothered; they were having so much fun and focused on their goals. For them, artificial nails weren't worth the trade-off.

While some of the girls in my school wore fake nails because they felt arti-ficial nails offered their own nails an added protection—because their own nails were either too weak or too brittle to withstand their lifestyle—most of the girls who wore fake nails did so because they felt artificial nails were the "in" thing to do. Natural nails will always be in vogue. If you look closely at the hands on the models in the top magazines, you'll notice that almost all of them wear short nails. Short nails that are well cared for are pretty nails. You can see my bias here: I'm making the case for wearing your own nails, and for wearing them at a length that looks nice and allows you to use your hands. This is not to say that you shouldn't apply artificial nails for those special occa-sions when you want your nails to be longer or more glamorous than the way you normally wear them. And this brings me to the second reason you probably don't want to wear fake nails. Your natural nails are porous, that means they need to breathe. When you cover—or rather smother—them with a layer of plastic or acrylic, the moisture that would normally evaporate is locked in. It doesn't take too long before the nail is saturated in its own moisture. This causes it to become soft, and as a result, it loosens from the nail bed. In a word, it is a ruined nail. The nail has been destroyed. Until it grows completely out, your nail is too soft to sustain itself. As a result, it chips and peels easily.

Wearing a covering over your own natural nail for so long—glues, adhesives, acrylic, plastic—is also why fake nails are associated with some nasty infections. There are of course some alternatives. Glue-ons and tips are great short-term remedies, especially for special occasions when you want to even out a broken nail (easy to do with glue-ons or just adding a tip), wear your nails longer than you normally do (easy to do with glue-ons or just adding tips), or want to have your nails decorated in a wildly fun sort of way (easy to do with glue-ons).

Options! Decisions! Choices! How do you decide? Here's the scoop on fake nails.

The Scoop on Nails: Acrylics, Wraps, Tips, Glue-Ons and More!

Whether you are just curious about artificial nails or choose to wear them because you feel your own nails are very soft or too brittle and believe that by wearing artificial nails, your own nails will have the time to "recover"—get longer, harder, stronger or whatever—the following information should prove useful in helping you make wise choices in the care of your nails.

- **Sculptured nails.** This process is best done in a salon. Most teens find it messy and very difficult to do for themselves. The process is this: A mold is placed over your own nail (this guides the shape). Next, layers of acrylic are brushed on until the desired length and thickness is achieved. The nails are then filed and polished (if not already pre-polished). As your natural nail grows, there will be a noticeable gap between your natural nail and the fake nail, so you have to return to the salon to get what is called a "refill," which is the filling in, or rather, covering up of the new portion of your natural nail so as to match your fake nail.

Upside: Sculptured nails are very realistic looking.

Downside: Sculptured nails are devastating to your natural nail. Precisely because acrylics stay so long—covering and smothering your natural nail—they saturate, soften and weaken the nail plate, and often completely destroy the nail bed below. Because acrylic is highly toxic material, it can irritate the cuticle as well as the skin surrounding the nail. Acrylics are notorious for causing serious nail infections. Expect to be in the salon an hour or longer. And they are expensive. Depending on the particular salon you use, getting acrylics can run anywhere between $20 and $80, and repairing them runs anywhere from $15 to $45, depending upon the number of damaged nails.

- **Wraps.** This is best left to a salon manicurist as well. The process is this: Strips of silk paper or linen are applied over your own natural nail and wrapped just under your own natural nail. They are then trimmed to size and glued on your nail. After this dries, the wrap is manicured like a natural nail.

    Upside: These nails will last anywhere from one to three weeks. Because your nail has been reinforced, your nails feel durable (especially if you considered your own natural nail weak).

    Downside: Because they stay on so long, they can soften and weaken the nail plate. They can cause infections. They can cause short-term and permanent damage to your nail. Expect to be in the salon an hour or longer. They are expensive.

- **Press-on nails.** You can buy these at beauty-supply stores and in most drugstores, even grocery stores. The process is this: Select the nails that appeal to you. Within the package of nails you should find an adhesive that is meant to be applied over your own nails (follow the specific directions contained in the package you purchase). Applying one nail at a time, press the fake nail over your own. Since you buy them in the length of your choice, you shouldn't have to cut or file these artificial nails. Some brand names offer the gel-adhesive already on the nail. With these, you simply peel back the protective coating and apply the fake nail to your own. Allow the specified time to dry so that it to adheres snuggly to your own nails.

    Upside: These plastic nails come in a wide variety of shapes, lengths and colors so you can readily change them as you wish. Because they don't stay on long (one to four days) there is less (if any) damage to your natural nail. They rarely cause infections. They are inexpensive.

    Downside: They don't look as natural as do, say, sculptured nails. They are known to pop off easily, so they aren't as dependable as some other artificial nails.

- **Nail tips.** These are made from acetate and can be applied at home or at a salon. The process is this: The acetate nail is selected to match the size and shape of your other nails. It is then cut and trimmed so that it matches perfectly. Then it is applied over the tips of your own nails and glued on with an acrylate adhesive. Next, a mixture of acrylic powder and glue is applied over your entire nail so that the nail tip looks like a natural extension of your own nail. Your nails are then polished in the color of your choice (even as a French manicure).

    Upside: They look natural. If overall your nails are in nice shape except for a nail or two that is broken, you can have a tip put on so that it matches the length of your other nails. And of course, you can have a tip applied to each of your nails. As a rule, most salons charge $3 a tip, and often a little less depending on how many you are having applied. Nail tips are easier to remove (they need to be soaked off with a special solution, though they can fall off from natural wear and tear).

Downside: Because nail tips don't really have much to hang on to—just the tip of your own finger, a very strong adhesive is used to glue them on. This adhesive is so strong that it is often associated with severe allergic reactions, especially if you put your fingers near your (sensitive) eyes.

Nail-care specialists confirm that in a great many cases, wearing artificial nails not only can cause infections, but also can damage your natural nails, even to the point where they never are as strong and healthy as they should be. You really have to ask yourself if it's worth wearing them.

Having Pretty Hands Is in Your Hands

Having beautiful hands and nails can give you added confidence in the way you present yourself, secure in knowing your hands are a spokeswoman of your good grooming—and good health! Like most things, having pretty hands is in *your* hands. [See colorplates 72–73.]

21

Fancy—and Comfortable—Feet

Make time away from highways and promises,
time for quiet, peace and love.

—PETER STONE

Putting Your Best Foot Forward:
Facts from a (Highly Paid) Foot Model

I have a good friend, Angeline D'iamto, who is a shoe model. Sounds like a great job doesn't it, getting paid big sums of money to model the latest and hottest fashion in shoe designs! But Angeline, like the rest of us, has got to do her homework. In her case, it's making sure her feet are in top-notch condition—or she won't be selected for a job.

Caring for your feet regularly throughout the year makes all the difference in looking great as well as in your sense of comfort—no matter if your feet are making their appearance for your eyes only, or if you're wearing bare feet in dress sandals to your boyfriend's sister's wedding. I asked Angeline to share her secrets for having beautiful feet. Here they are:

- Wear comfortable shoes, which means wear "flats"—shoes without heels—even to dress-up events!
- Apply Vaseline to your feet and wear socks to bed every night—even in the summer!
- Get a pedicure every ten days.
- Exfoliate your feet every other week.
- If you must wear high heels, limit the amount of time you spend standing in them.
- Never get athlete's foot!

Are you surprised at how commonsense these tips are? All of them are easy for any of us to follow.

Hazardous High Heels: Comfort Counts!

When I was a sophomore, I was asked out by a guy who was a senior. He had dated a really pretty and feminine girl who always dressed nicely. Several months after they broke up, he asked me out. He was a neat guy and a popular one. I was flattered. I can't tell you how much I waited and waited for the day of our date!

As soon as he asked me out, I got busy thinking about and shopping for just the right things to wear on that first date. My goal was to look good—well actually, my goal was to look drop-dead gorgeous. And I did. From a great outfit to the most incredibly dainty, strapping three-inch sandals, I was smashing! The problem was, my toes were getting a smashing, too. Before my new love and I had even arrived at the restaurant, the little straps cut into my feet. By the time dessert was served, the hollows of my feet were burning so badly, I could hardly concentrate on what my date was talking about. And I never did make it through more than one hour of dancing before I simply didn't care what he was talking about, even though he was whispering sweet nothings in my ear! I simply had to get out of those strappy little sandals before I was going to faint from the pain of them.

Do you own a pair of shoes that feel like a torture device after spending a few hours walking, dancing or even just standing in them? Most of us girls do. Think of those flashy and adorable spiked heels with the pointy toes and flashy straps that looked gorgeous with your prom dress—you know the ones—you carried them out the door as you hobbled from the gym after a couple hours of dancing in them. I've learned to wear comfortable shoes. Especially these days when I'm doing workshops and seminars and am on my feet for hours at a time, and sometimes for a full day. When my feet hurt, I hurt all over. My foot-modeling friend made it perfectly clear that comfort counts for her, too. She *always* wears comfortable shoes.

Foot specialists, known as *podiatrists,* agree that wearing comfortable shoes, ones that fit well and don't have a high heel, is always the best thing you can do for your feet. Even if you adjust to the discomfort of high heels and narrow toes today, there's still a price to pay in the damage they can do to the health of your feet in the future. From pain to deformities, the shoes we wear do more damage than the wear and tear we put our feet through.

My foot-model friend says she wears low heels no matter how formal the occasion. If you've got a closet filled with hazardous heels, you'll want to limit your standing time in them. If you're going out on a big date that includes dinner at a nice restaurant and a play, you might decide to go ahead and wear your heels. If you'll be dancing or doing a lot of walking, better take along a backup pair for comfort. If you'd rather be comfortable than carting along a second pair of shoes, wear a pair that can take you through the entire evening in ease. Enjoy yourself—go for comfort.

How to "Shed" the Skin on Your Feet

Rough, dry and broken skin on your feet can be anything but attractive. In earlier chapters you've learned about exfoliating the skin on your face and your body. You can also exfoliate the skin on your feet, adding to their beauty—and to your comfort. Exfoliating the skin on your feet can prevent dry layers of skin from building up and becoming callused.

Okay, so your boyfriend is going to hold your hand, not your foot— although many a boyfriend of mine rubbed my feet as a sweet gesture, especially when at times the two of us would be sitting on the couch watching television. There were times when I was more than happy to leave my socks on—because of the shape my toes or feet were in. And, there were other times when I was more than happy to remove my socks and let my pretty and soft feet be romanced.

How do you keep your feet smooth and soft? Like Angeline you can wear Vaseline and socks to bed every night—even in the summer! If the skin on your feet is really dry and cracks easily, before you go to bed try massaging your feet with a moisturizing cream that has emollients and then cover them up with socks overnight. This keeps the moisture in and warms it up so that it does a deeper job of soothing and smoothing your feet. Angeline uses a mixture of sugar and olive oil on her feet after showers. After smoothing this mixture into her feet, she rinses them and then pats them dry. I tried this little secret of hers myself and found that it really did make my feet feel velvety. Try it for yourself.

Pampered with a Pedicure

A good pedicure after you've washed your feet is the epitome of being pampered, and it assures that your feet will look their very best. But a pedicure, like a manicure, is also important to nail and health care. While we may not need (or be able to afford) a weekly pedicure, it's a good idea to have one every ten days to two weeks. Pedicures are expensive for most teens; a typical pedicure costs about fifteen to twenty-five dollars. Good news: You don't need big money to get weekly pedicures, you can do them yourself.

Because a pedicure is like a manicure, about taking care of nail health, and because painting your toes is much the same process, I'll let some of the photos in this section do the talking and instead provide you with some very important tips for doing your pedicure.

Terrific Toe Tips

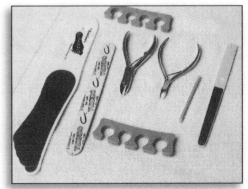

- Do dry off thoroughly. After bathing or showering always completely dry your feet and between each toe with a towel. This helps prevent fungal infections.
- Do get the proper pedicure tools, and do clean them with soap and water or with anti-bacterial spray or isopropyl rubbing alcohol before and after each pedicure.
- Immediately following a shower or bath, push back cuticles, and use a pumice stone to smooth away calluses or to remove dead skin cells.
- Don't cut your nails when they are wet or damp. Wet nails are more prone to tearing.

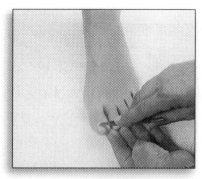

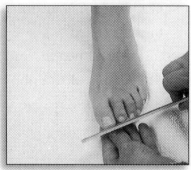

- Don't use cuticle nippers to cut your nails or you'll end up with torn nails (and dull nippers).
- Don't cut your nails too short; short nails are more prone to becoming ingrown. It's best to cut them blunt, then file them so they are straight across.
- Do use an emery board to shape your nails (a metal file can weaken them).
- Never use a razor to remove calluses and corns. Instead see a foot specialist or your family doctor. He or she will know the best way to treat these conditions. (This is especially the case should you suffer from an ingrown nail, or should you have developed a really bad blister that becomes infected.)

Polished Pretty Policies

You can polish your toenails like a pro. Here's how:

- Turn the polish bottle upside down and roll it from side to side rather than shaking it, which can make bubbles in it.
- Sit on a chair with your knees close to your chest. Use the hand you aren't polishing with to hold the toe you are painting.
- Before applying polish, clean the excess from the side of the brush that you won't be using. On the side that you are using, leave polish on half of the brush for the big toe and just on the tip for the little ones.
- If you are right-handed, start polishing on your left foot, from pinkie to big toe; on your right foot, from big toe to pinkie. Lefties should work right to left.

- Wait two to three minutes between coats to prevent streaking. The more coats you apply, the longer each will take to dry. Painting nails before bed is not such a good idea because nail polish takes a long time to set and when your nails come in contact with the sheet, it dulls the appearance of the glossy look you were trying to achieve.

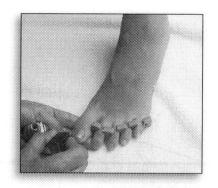

- Re-dip the nail-polish brush before painting each nail, so polish doesn't have time to dry on the brush and cause streaking.

- For a fast, long-lasting pedicure, use light, frosted nail colors—mistakes and chipping won't be obvious.

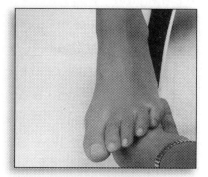

- Prolong the life of your pedicure by applying base coat and one coat of color the first day, a second coat two days later, and top-coat whenever you need to revive the shine. Using fewer coats reduces the chances of chipping.

- If you don't have time for polish, use a nail buffer to smooth and shine the surface of the nail, then apply a dab of nail oil.

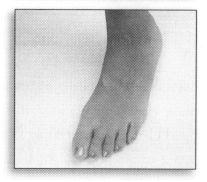

There's a Fungus Among Us: Athlete's Foot!

As Angeline says, the worst thing that can happen to her job-wise is that she come down with not a sore throat, but a foot fungus. Athlete's foot may not be the occupational disaster for you that it is for my friend the foot model, but you certainly want to do all you can to avoid it!

Athlete's foot is a common fungal infection that causes burning, itching, cracking and peeling of the skin on the bottom of the foot and between the toes. It's definitely a "no" to having clean and beautiful feet. To prevent it, keep your feet dry and wear absorbent cotton socks. No matter how good your friend's intention in offering to loan you a pair, avoid sharing socks. Also avoid sharing washcloths and towels. Sprinkle your soles and between your toes with powder in the morning to help prevent athlete's foot and other types of fungus. The bad news is that athlete's foot won't go away on its own. The good news is that there are medications that can control the infection, so if you do get it, go to a drugstore and ask the pharmacist to recommend the "latest and best cure." If you develop a severe case, by all means, see a foot doctor or your family doctor.

"Toe" Your Weight!

From comfortable shoes to protecting your feet against fungus, from trimming your toenails to painting them in a pretty shade of polish, all are about head-to-toe beauty. Your care and attention to this beauty "footwork" assures you a better chance for healthy, attractive feet. As you know, healthy feet are happy feet!

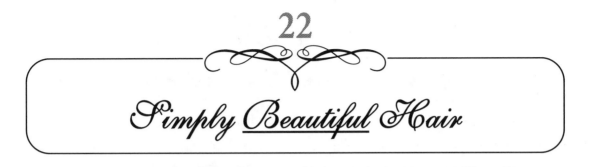

22

Simply Beautiful Hair

*Nothing is so commonplace as
to wish to be remarkable.*

—Oliver Wendell Holmes Jr.

Hair with a Reputation

A good friend of mine, Michelle Geller, has exquisitely beautiful hair. It's long, thick, lustrous and cut in a style that frames her face in a most flattering way. It's so well-kept that your eyes are just instantly drawn to it. In fact, Michelle's hair is so dazzling that she's become known by it, a point that became clear one day when one of the girls at school commented that Lane Thomas—a really cool senior at our school—had asked Michelle to the spring dance. "Who is Michelle?" one of the girls in our group inquired, only to be informed, "You know, that girl with the *really* beautiful hair!"

"Oh, yeah, her!" came the first girl's instant reply. While not everyone in our school knew Michelle personally, almost all of us could identify who she was at the mention of her lustrous hair.

Mane Advice:
How to Have Beautiful Hair

As her friends found out, dazzling hair makes a lasting impression. In fact, beautiful hair has so much sex appeal that at first glance, we often describe someone as "attractive" by mere virtue of the overall glamour of her hair.

What makes for beautiful hair? For starters, luster, that glossy look that we associate with healthy, vibrant hair. But glossy hair is more a by-product of being undamaged: When the outer layer of a strand of hair, the *cuticle,* has suffered no damage (from sun, blow-drying, rollers) and is naturally well-oiled, it's smooth and even. As such, it is a surface that reflects the light; it shines. On the other hand, should the surface of your hair strand be damaged—because it is not getting adequate natural oils or is overly dry—then the surface of the hair splits apart, looking dull or in poor condition. Certain shampoos and conditioners can temporarily add shine and lustre to your hair by filling in the cracks and tears to the surface of the strand, but they cannot repair your damaged hair. (Setting lotions, gels, mousses, hairsprays and dyes leave a residue on your hair that can also make it appear dull.)

Again, hair that is not damaged is beautiful hair. And of course, volume, a good cut and a style that works for your face are also essentials to a beautiful mane. Here are some very important "beauty treatments" on how you can have great hair.

Beauty Treatment # 1: Groom from the Inside

Good grooming certainly plays a big role in having great hair, but perhaps more than the color, cut or style, beautiful hair's first beauty treatment begins from the inside out. Again, diet, rest, exercise and drinking plenty of water are important to being healthy. Hair follicles are nourished by the foods you eat—your diet.

As important as good grooming is, my hair is always at its "best" during those times when my diet is good and when I stick to a regime of regularly working out and getting the sleep I need. Drinking plenty of water is important, too. When I don't do these things, and when I splurge on foods such as hamburgers, French fries and chocolate, not only is my hair greasy and less manageable, it lacks shine and doesn't have the vibrancy it normally does. Just as our hair is susceptible to the elements to which it is exposed, humidity for example, it is sensitive to what's going on inside. Contrary to what you read on many of the hair-care products, your hair cannot be "invigorated" or "rejuvenated" from the outside. You may put additives on your hair that will give it shine and make it appear more full (though some products, as well as exposure to the elements or even illness, can cause your hair to be overly dry and brittle and break off) but nothing will "feed" it or make it grow. All that happens from the inside out. This is because your hair is a nonliving fibrous protein (keratin). The hair root, however, is alive, and is nourished not from the outside, but, rather, from the inside.

Beauty Treatment # 2: Wash It

Cleanliness is not only a first impression of your hair's beauty—but of you, too. When you see someone who doesn't keep her hair clean, do you wonder if she took a shower, or brushed her teeth, or . . . ? No doubt about it. Clean hair is a real positive in your appearance.

How often should you wash your hair? It depends. Not everyone needs to wash her hair every day, particularly girls of color. Many African American girls tell me their hair tends to be on the dry side and needs to be washed less frequently. While it's important to have clean hair, you can overdo it. If you have very oily hair, you probably need to wash your hair every day. If you have normal to dry hair, you only need to wash your hair every other day, maybe even every third day. Too much washing will wash out the natural oils in your hair, oils that are needed to keep your hair strong and healthy. Then your hair is dry, looks dull and lacks luster. You will have to monitor this for yourself based on your hair type and how often it needs shampooing to feel clean and look its best. Again, hair type is important. Girls of color, for example, usually have a far different hair type than girls of European descent, but even so, hair type is not so cut and dried, as you'll see in this section. Luckily, there are many hair-care products on the market designed with our individual needs in mind. You can find an assortment of hair-care products in most drug stores and beauty-supply stores. Should you have questions about which products are best for you or how they should be used, sales clerks at beauty supply stores are a good source of information because not only do they hear about the product from the manufacturer, they also hear what does and doesn't work from their other customers. And of course, a visit to a hair salon for a consultation with someone trained in hair care can prove useful in helping you determine your hair type as well as the best ways to care for your particular hair.

Is There a "Best" Shampoo?

There are many shampoos on the market. If you compare a handful of hair-care products, you will notice that while packaging and cost vary a great deal (expensive does not always mean better), most of the products contain many of the same basic ingredients, but there are some differences. So read the label before you choose a product. The first rule is to choose a shampoo according to your hair type: dry, oily or normal. The bottle will say, "for dry hair," or "for moderate to oily hair." If you can't tell if your hair is oily or dry, it probably isn't

either. Hair-care experts say a simple way to determine your hair type is to pluck out a single strand
of hair. Holding this strand between both hands,
pull it apart. If it snaps easily, your hair is either fine
or oily. If the strand is hard to break, it means your
hair is either coarse or dry. If you still can't tell the
difference, schedule a consultation with a hair-care
expert at a beauty salon to advise you as to the con-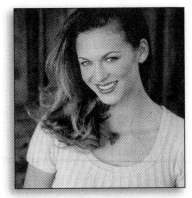
dition of your hair, as well as suggest the best way for you to care for your hair.
You may be surprised at what you find out. For example, perhaps you use hairspray and mousse on a daily basis and because of the sticky buildup (residue)
you wash your hair every day. As a result, your hair is dry. Because your hair is
dry, and because you wash it daily, you think you should use a mild, moisturizing shampoo so as not to make it any dryer than it already is. But consider
that perhaps you are adding to the problem by over-washing your hair. A hair-
care specialist may very well advice to you forget the mild moisturizing shampoo and instead use a stronger one so that you can wash your hair less
frequently in order to give your hair and scalp the chance to rehydrate between
washings. Or, if you have extremely dry hair or your hair splits easily, you may
be advised to use a special conditioner as opposed to changing your shampoo.
Should your hair be damaged from products with chemicals designed to
straighten or dye your hair, you may be advised that the "magic cure" is a shampoo (as in protein-enriched shampoo) versus a conditioner. Again, a professional can help you decide what is best for you, including suggesting the best
comb or brushes that work best with your hair type.

And there is something else you need to consider. Just because you are in
the habit of buying shampoo for, let's say, dry hair, don't assume it will always
be dry. If you observe closely, there are times when your hair type changes.
For example, it may be more oily during your menstrual cycle than the other

twenty-five days of the month. And, depending on the season—and most especially if you live in climates where you have a hot or cold season followed by a wet season—you may need to vary your shampoo from time to time. Regardless of the seasons and changes in environments, however (and even if your hair is naturally oily), always buy hair-care products that are alcohol-free. Alcohol dries out your hair and scalp and can contribute to dandruff and other scalp problems.

With all the shampoo products on the market, it can be confusing knowing what to buy. Don't just grab the first one on the shelf, and don't just buy the one with the pretty packaging. And unless the one you've been using works just fine for you, the next time you are ready to purchase a shampoo, stop and read the label carefully. You may have to experiment with a couple kinds of shampoo, but it's worth it. And of course, depending on your hair care needs, you may need a couple of different kinds. I use three different shampoos, depending on what condition my hair is in.

Basically, there are two types of shampoo: cleansing shampoo and conditioning shampoo. The difference is this: *Cleansing shampoos* contain additives that are designed to clean your hair, to remove hair oils and strip off the buildup left by hairsprays, mousse, gels or other hair-care products (but not *permanent* dyes). *Conditioning shampoos* have additives designed to improve the *appearance* of the outer structure of your hair and make it easier to style. Whereas a cleansing shampoo is pretty straightforward, you will find there are a number of additives in the conditioning shampoos, all supposedly designed to do various things. The following profile on shampoos can help you sort out what may work best and when:

- **Protein-enriched shampoo.** Sometimes you will see these advertised as pH-balanced. These are formulas designed to improve damaged hair. Hair-care experts say they work because they are designed to coat the damaged hair and fill in the cracks or split ends, making the hair appear more full. And, hair that is smooth reflects the light, so this product would also make your hair have luster, shine. If your hair is badly damaged (especially if the tips are split or frayed) you may want to try a product that is protein enriched.

- **Moisturizing shampoo.** These products are designed to trap moisture in the hair strands, thus preventing them from drying out. If you have normally dry hair (or limp hair) or if you spend a great deal of time outside in the elements, a moisturizing shampoo might be right for you.
- **Balsam shampoo.** Balsam (sometimes advertised as body-building shampoo) is an additive that strengthens and thickens the hair. It does this by restoring the damaged shaft. If you have very fine or limp hair or simply want the look of fuller hair, you may want to try a conditioning shampoo with this additive.
- **Herbal shampoo.** These are designed to soften the hair, make it manageable and to intensity its color. Ingredients such as aloe, honey and vitamins are all promoted to be spectacular for your hair. The hair-care experts I checked with said that while ingredients such as these make the product sound wonderfully useful, they couldn't vouch for them doing what they say they will—though they do add to the expense of the product. Again, you can't feed the hair from the outside. It's an inside-out job! One additive is worth special consideration, however, and that is sunscreen ingredients, such as cinnamates and PABA. We often forget that the UV rays can take their toll on hair, but they do. I suggest that you always look for these additives in any hair-care product.

The best, basic advice on shampooing is this:

- If your hair is normal or normally oily, try a cleansing shampoo.
- If your hair is dry, brittle, sun damaged or dyed or bleached, try a pH-balanced shampoo.
- If your hair is limp, thin or exceptionally thin, try a body-building shampoo.
- If you have a special condition, such as dandruff, or if you have picked

up a case of head lice, buy a shampoo specifically advertised to go to work on the problem you are addressing. If you are following the directions and the shampoo isn't resolving the problem, see your family doctor or a dermatologist. At the very least, go see your school nurse or tell your parents. It's important to treat these conditions. Always do those things that protect your health and well-being.

Here are some other tips on washing your hair:

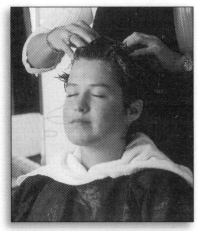

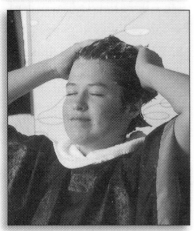

- Unless your hair is really oily or unless you use hairspray, spritz and other hair-care products on a daily basis, *you do not need to apply shampoo more than once* when you wash your hair.
- Since shampoo can dry out the tips of your hair, apply the shampoo mainly to the roots and the scalp.
- Hot water is drying to your hair, so avoid using very hot water when you wash it.
- Make sure you rinse your hair thoroughly after shampooing. Because of its drying effect, you want to be sure all soap is rinsed out.
- Use the coolest water you can tolerate for the final rinse. In addition to stimulating the circulation in the scalp, cool water will close the hair cuticle, which prevents the ends of your hair from looking split and frizzy.

Oily Bangs?

Don't assume that if your bangs are oily it means that the rest of your hair needs washing. If you wear bangs and your face has a tendency to be oily (or your bangs or strands along your face are oily because of contact with your makeup), it's possible that only your bangs and the strands of hair along your face need washing. Wash your bangs with a wet washcloth using only a tiny dab of shampoo. Rinse them thoroughly. Apply a conditioner only if your hair is thin and you need it for control.

Beauty Treatment # 3: Condition It

In most cases you want to add a conditioner to your hair after shampooing. However, if you have problems with acne, you should be aware that conditioners can cause or aggravate breakouts. This is because it rubs off on your pillowcase and then gets on your face while you sleep. So if you are acne-prone, you may want to skip conditioning. (If you are unsure what to do or have other questions, ask a dermatologist.) Conditioner smoothes the hair and makes it easier to comb so that it doesn't break off while brushing. It also provides added protection against blow-drying and hot rollers, as well as protection from the elements, such as the sun.

If you look closely at conditioning hair-care products, you'll notice that some are called "creme rinse" while others are labeled "conditioner." Both smooth and soften the hair and make it more manageable. The basic difference between a creme rinse and a conditioner is this:

- Creme rinse will provide a *light* conditioning, add shine and also detangle the hair so it is easier to brush while wet.
- A conditioner is more concentrated than creme rinse and is also more

penetrating. Conditioners relax the hair to make it softer and more manageable and give it shine.

Almost all conditioners require that you rinse your hair thoroughly after you've left them on your hair for three to ten minutes. Others are to be left on your hair and do not require that you rinse them out. If your hair is very dry, I would suggest that you look for a conditioner to leave in your hair (especially if you swim in chlorinated pools). Doing this can give you extra protection from the elements.

How to Select a Conditioner

A conditioner, like shampoo, should be selected according to your hair type, such as whether your hair is normal, dry or oily. You especially need to condition your hair if it is naturally dry or dried out due to overexposure from the sun, the cold or from swimming in chlorinated pools. After restoring moisture to your hair, you can go for the pizzazz: the conditioner advertising "adds body," "adds shine," or "for limp hair," "for fine hair," and so on.

Experiment with the products until you find those that work for you.

Beauty Treatment # 4: Go Easy on the Blow-Dryer

Blow-dryers, hot rollers and crimping and curling irons can dry your hair, as well as can cause split ends, and make your hair brittle, even break off. This is true for blow-drying your hair, especially if you do it often and use dryers higher than 1,400 or 1,600 watts. Almost all of the girls I know own a metal core brush to speed up the drying of their hair. If you do this, use it only when you have to, like at those times when you are running late and need to get going. But don't use it on a daily basis.

Here are some tips to avoid ruining your hair:

- Try using a low setting on your dryer, and always use a diffuser (a little gadget that attaches to the hairdryer and spreads the air with less force) so the heat damage to the hair is minimized.
- When possible, let your hair dry naturally, particularly on the weekends or whenever you have the time to let it dry naturally.
- If you're looking for more volume in hair, a vent brush will help; for extra lift, hold your head upside down while you're blow-drying it.

Beauty Treatment # 5:
Then and Wow! Choose a Hairstyle That's Right for You

Your hairstyle can dramatically change the way you look, as you can see in the computer-generated photographs of me [see next page and colorplates 57–71]. Sometimes it's difficult to tell what you would look like with a certain style. There are two ways to check out how you would look before going and getting a cut, getting a new style, or even adding streaks or coloring. First, you can try on a wig before taking any big step. When you do this, use a full-length mirror to analyze the prospective new look from every angle so you can better judge the proper proportion of your hair to your individual shape. Another way to test a style is to call a salon that uses a video-imaging system to superimpose your face on different hairstyles and in different colors. Some salons will do this as a complimentary service they offer. Others charge a nominal fee ($20 to $40 is the average).

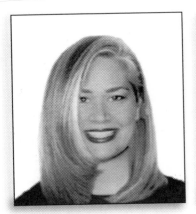
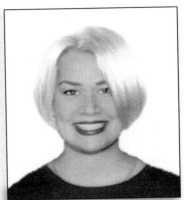
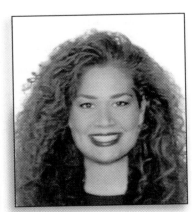

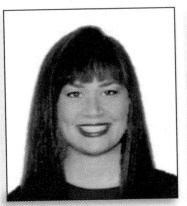
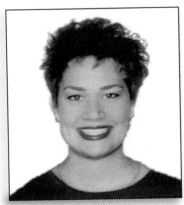
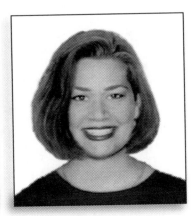

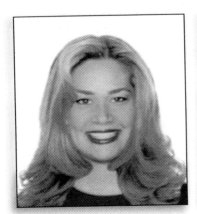
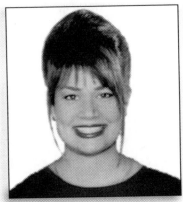
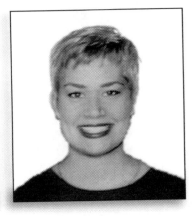

The photos of me are computer-generated by Susan Gilbert of New Looks on Video. Video-imaging is a great idea because in addition to seeing what hairstyle and what length of hair looks best on you, you can also see what you would look like with black hair or as a brunette, a redhead or blonde. If a picture is worth a thousand words, it might also save you the expense (and heartache) of a haircut (or coloring) that, in the long run, is not really right for you. Judging from the series of images of me by New Looks on Video [see previous page and colorplates 57–71], which color and style do you think is best for me?

The most important consideration in choosing a hairstyle is that it flatter your features—and, of course, that you like it. Here are some other suggestions for finding a style that's right for you:

- Start by looking around at other people's hair. Look around and notice the styles others are wearing.

- When you see someone with a style you like, observe the person for a moment. Does the style look and "feel" like one you could wear? I remember seeing a woman with a style that I thought was really cool and sexy. It was a wedge over one eye, and then I realized the woman had to keep swinging her head from side to side to remove the hair from her eyes. After several moments of observing the woman, I knew for certain that the same hairstyle on me would drive me positively crazy.

- Spend some time looking through magazines seeing the different possibilities, seeing what you like. You might even ask your friends if they think a certain style would look good on you. And, of course, looking at the images of hairstyles on me, could you see yourself wearing any of them?

- Get a professional's opinion. Make an appointment specifically to get advice. Ask a hairstylist what style he or she would suggest, and why.

Does Your Hairstyle Flatter Your Features?

The hair style you choose should take into consideration the size and shape of your face and features. Michelle complained that her forehead was too high, but you would never know it because she wore bangs that flattered this feature.

Isn't it nice we girls have so many options with our hair! Like Michelle, who wore her hair in a style that flattered her best features, the right hairstyle can help you play down those things you don't like and accentuate your more flattering features. The following are just a few of the many suggestions I got from my friend Raymond David Farmer, a salon owner and popular stylist in my town.

- **Your jaw is square.** You can flatter it with a hairstyle that is swept back at the temples. This can be either a short cut that feathers down the neck, or a longer cut that is angled and ends below your chin.
- **Your forehead is narrow.** Backcomb the top to make your forehead appear wider.
- **Your forehead is really high.** You can fill it in with either a few wisps of bangs or full bangs, or an off-center part with some of your hair falling across the side of your forehead.
- **Your neck is short.** A short haircut will create the illusion of a longer neck. Highlights in your hair can draw attention to the hair and not the neck. No bangs.
- **Your chin is long.** You can balance it with a haircut that ends at your chin and is rounded and full.
- **Your chin is small.** You can enhance it with a hairstyle that ends either above or well below chin length, while also being cut to give you height at the crown.

The important thing is that you have well-groomed hair, and that you really like the way it looks on you.

Beauty Treatment # 6:
Scissor Sizzle—Get a Great Haircut

It's probably not wise to trust your haircut to a best friend, brother or younger sister, and you know what happens when your mom says she'll snip "only the dead ends." It's about as disastrous as when you trim it yourself. My suggestion is save up your money and let a professional do it for you. How do you find a good stylist? Referral is always a good place to start. Also, if someone has a hairstyle that you just love, whether it's someone you know or not, it's okay to ask them where they get it done. It's a compliment; most people won't mind your asking.

Here are helpful hints:

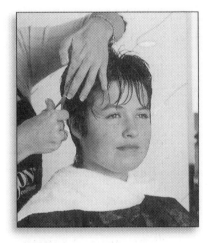

- **Do your homework before you walk into the hair salon.** Have an idea of what style you want. Bring a picture of the hairstyle with you or a composite of a couple of styles you like (such as the bangs on one model and the length of hair on another).

- **This is not the time to be shy.** Explain exactly how you would like your hair. Ask the stylist if you are making yourself clear. Don't assume that you are. Kindly ask if he or she would discuss with you his or her opinion as to whether or not it's a style for you.

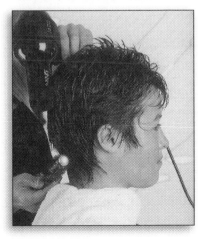

- **At your appointment say, "Please, no surprises."** Agree beforehand on exactly the length you want and watch carefully.

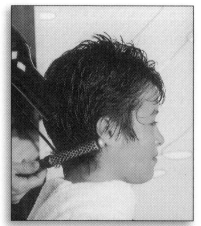

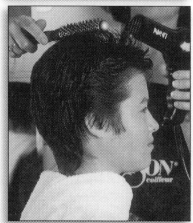

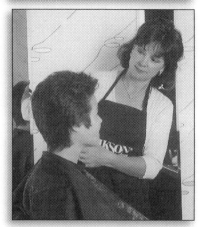

Hairstylist Michele Heppner and teen client

There's nothing worse than a hairstyle or a cut that is not what you want. Pay close attention to what the stylist is doing so that you can tell him or her not to go any shorter, or to take off a little more. Some people complain after they've left the salon, but say nothing while their hair is being cut. Don't let this happen to you. It's your hair and if you feel like most people, your hair is a large part of your identity.

- **Hold still while your bangs are being cut.** Stylists say it's even wise not to smile while your bangs are being cut because in smiling you raise your forehead and it makes the bangs come out shorter than you want them. So sit up straight, and during the time your bangs are being cut hold your smile.

- **Observe how your stylist is styling your hair** (rather than reading a magazine or listening in on a conversation going on in the chair beside you). Ask the stylist why he or she is using a particular size or style of brush, styling with a certain styling product or hair-spray, and so on.

- **After you've had a cut or style, ask how to maintain your new style,** or how to brush and dry your hair so it falls in place the way you want it to. Also ask her to suggest the best comb, brush and hair-care products to maintain your new style.

- **Ask questions about your hair.** For example, if you have a cowlick and are unable to tame it by blow-drying it in the opposite direction it grows, ask your hairdresser to apply a perm solution to the roots that will keep it in check. Ask about how to cure frizzy hair, control hair static other than by using hairspray before you brush it, and other things you would like him or her to help troubleshoot.

Beauty Treatment # 7:
Color Clarity—Highlighting and Coloring Your Hair

If you are going to color your hair—whether to just a shade darker or lighter than your natural color, or wanting to try chartreuse or lime-green—my suggestion is, don't do it yourself. Every day I see teens who have done their own coloring, and usually it's a disaster. Save up your money and have a professional do it. You can really damage your hair if you don't consider the condition your hair is in, and how it will respond to the chemicals in the coloring you're adding. Getting your hair colored in a salon is expensive, but if you shop around and compare, you're sure to find a salon that can do it for you and keep within your budget.

If going all the way with color is too much for you, you might try highlighting your hair. Highlights are always a nice touch, and give you an entirely new and fresh look. Here are a few good rules to keep in mind before you do:

- Adding a few subtle highlights to the sides of your face and your bangs can brighten your complexion.
- If you have brown or dark-blonde hair, for a soft and natural look, choose amber or gold streaks.
- If your hair is auburn, for a soft and natural look, choose strawberry or gold streaks.

- Never put highlights too closely together or they won't look natural.
- When you apply highlights, if you brush along the curve of the cut, your hair will look fuller and thicker.
- Once you've colored, avoid hot oil treatments because hot oils strip color. Do, however, use a conditioner on a regular basis.

Can You Make Your Hair Grow Faster?

No, you can't, unfortunately. I've checked with the experts and there are simply no reliable products that act as a "fertilizer" to make your hair grow. This is because the part of your hair that you see (the *shaft*) is a nonliving entity (it's made up of keratin). The part responsible for hair growth is the live cells that are deep within the root. At the root level, a hair shaft is created and starts its journey toward becoming your mane.

The process for hair growth is relatively predetermined. Your hair grows in cycles, known as the growing, resting and falling out phase. *The growing phase* is roughly two to five years for healthy hair. During this phase, fresh keratin is released from the root into the strand of hair and thus keeps it growing (½ inch to 1 inch per month is the norm). The growing phase is followed by a *resting phase*, believed to be only a three- to four-week cycle, before the falling out phase begins. The *falling out* phase lasts somewhere between two and five months, during which time a single strand of hair sheds and is replaced by a new one from the same hair follicle.

Luckily, each hair follicle is independent of the others, each one having their own little calendar to adhere to. This way, we don't shed all of our hair at one time—or else there would be remittent periods when we would each be bald!

But even if you can't make your hair grow faster than it does, as you learned in this chapter, there are ways to care for it so it doesn't get overly dry and brittle and break off easily (such as protecting it from the damaging effects of the sun, hair dryers and harsh products).

Wigging Out: Ways to Change Your Style

Hair extensions are really costly, but for special occasions, they can be a great way to add intrigue and pizzazz to your look. The application of hair extensions is very specialized: Every salon doesn't offer them and every hairstylist doesn't have the training to apply them. So, you'll have to find a salon that's equipped to offer hair extensions. They're very expensive, but, most likely, you'd be getting them for a special photo or special occasion. Again, ask around, explain exactly what you want and get an estimate of the charges before you schedule an appointment.

You can also wear a wig. Women have been wearing wigs for years, and while I don't suggest you wear a wig all day long, some wigs are lightweight, allow your head to breathe, and look like a real head of hair and not a "wig." I especially like former model and now clothing- and wig-designer Cheryl Tiegs's line of wigs. My natural hair is auburn brown and I like to wear it long and straight, so I purchased a shorter styled wig. I don't wear the wig very often, but when I do, I really like the way it looks and feels. I paid about $120 for mine, which is in the moderate to moderately high range. Prices vary, according to whether the wig is made of human hair or synthetic hair.

Because I love to wear my hair long, for me, a short wig is a nice alternative, one that I didn't think I'd try but now that I have, I really like. You may, too, especially if your hair is very slow-growing and there are times you want longer hair, or want to wear a style that is completely different in color or length than your own.

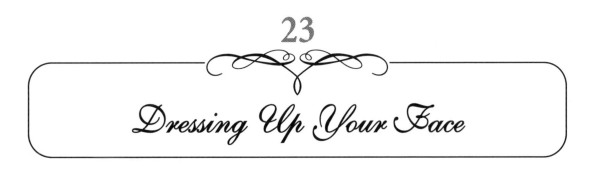

23

Dressing Up Your Face

*Ah, but a man's reach should exceed his grasp
—or what's a heaven for?*

—Robert Browning

The Face: The Artist's Canvas

Self-confidence, goals, family and friends, a way with color and style—you're well on your way to feeling great and looking hot! As if you need more!

But there is more! With a mere wave of the magic wand—the makeup wand, that is—you can appease the Cinderella in you, and become the Cinderella *of your choice* by defining how you'd like to present yourself to the world—and on any given day! Not every girl wears makeup and certainly not everyone wears it all the time. Some girls opt to wear only a light powder, lip gloss and little mascara, a perfect and simple everyday look, especially for school. Some girls go all out, and sometimes that's nice, too. And of course, sometimes, it's too much for an on-the-job occasion such as school.

For special events you definitely want to go "high glamour." No problem, you can up your level of "pizzazz" with the stroke of a brush! How fun. And practical, too.

Just as magic creates an illusion, so can makeup. I'm sure you've looked at before-and-after photos of models, some of which caused you to stand back and say, "Wow! Can you believe it's the same person?" Whether you want to simply enhace your look—or dramatically change it—you can. Selecting the right kinds of products for your skin and the shades that work best for you—along with applying them skillfully—is the real magic in makeup.

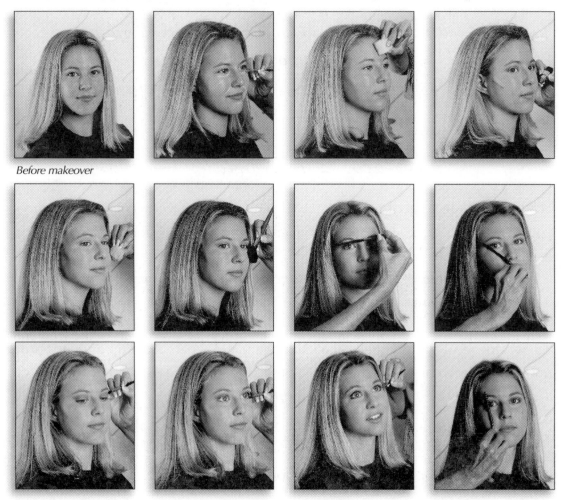

Before makeover

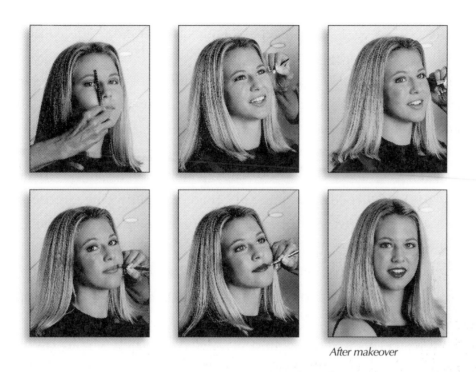

After makeover

Beauty Step # 1: Artful Applications—Foundation

Has anyone ever told you that you looked "different" not just because you were wearing makeup, but wearing the right makeup, artfully applied, for your skin type? Both make a big difference. If you've ever just slathered on your makeup because you've been in a big hurry (or borrowed makeup from a friend), you maybe noticed that just because you were wearing makeup didn't mean you looked "better."

Choosing the right cosmetics is important. So is their artful application, as you will see illustrated in the colorplates of makeup artist Lois Pearl applying makeup to teen Carrie Hague [see photos here and colorplates 76–93].

Your face is your canvas. Just as an artist prepares a canvas before putting the painting on it, you need to prepare your face for makeup. To do so, use a base makeup called foundation. Foundation, which is usually a lightweight cream with color, can mask the little blotches and color variations in your face, and make your skin look smooth and soft. Here are some tips for choosing the best foundation for you.

- Choose the makeup that is right for your skin type. If your skin tends to be oily, choose *water-based* cosmetics. If your skin is on the dry side, use *oil-based* cosmetics. If your skin is normal to slightly oily, choose *powder-based* cosmetics. Powder tones down shine, but be aware that powder-based makeups may contain oil, so if you are acne-prone it may not be the best choice for you. If your skin is very oily or if you are acne-prone, choose an *oil-free* makeup (these are usually alcohol- or glycerin-based products).

- Sample testers in a store to find a color that matches your own natural coloring. You want foundation to be the same as your skin tone. Don't use foundation to change your face's color. For example, if you are naturally pale, foundation is not supposed to give you a golden tan (you can use artificial tanning products for that). Ask the salesclerk to help you find a shade that works for you. Often, she will apply a dab to the inside of your wrist, and have you blend it in. If you can't see the color, it's probably the right shade for you.

- Don't confuse foundation with corrective concealer. If you have acne, or even just a few assorted pimples, treat them with a special product, a corrective concealer, before you apply your foundation. Makeup experts will tell you that green is the best color for camouflaging inflamed skin, such as acne—zits. Yellow will also work, and has a more natural looking tone to it. To use, apply the corrective concealer, and then use your regular foundation over it. Go light on the corrective concealer; too much makeup over a skin bump will make it appear even more obvious. And by the way, you can use the same corrective concealer to cover freckles, moles or a birthmark.

- Choose a foundation that has an SPF (sun protection factor) to protect your face from the sun. These foundations give you extra protection against burning and chapping, and hold in moisture to keep your skin soft.

Using a Concealer

A concealer is a form of makeup specially designed to conceal, for example, if you want to lighten up under the eye area, or you want to minimize the appearance of a blemish. Concealer goes on before your foundation. Use a brush to apply your concealer. Put it only in those places where you want to lighten up, such as under the eye area, or to cover blotches or skin discol- 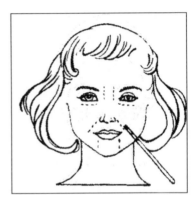 orations. (If you use it all over, your makeup will look and feel like pancake syrup on your face.)

How to Apply Foundation

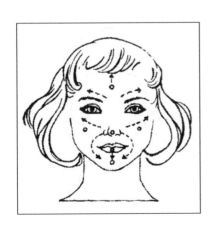 The art to applying foundation is to dab it on gently, on your forehead, cheeks, nose and chin. Smooth the makeup evenly over your face, stroking gently in the directions shown in the diagram.

The foundation should be blended only to your jawline. The skin on your neck and the skin on your face are slightly different colors, so putting the foundation on your neck won't look natural. Smooth the foundation carefully along the jaw-line (or you may look as if you are wearing a mask!).

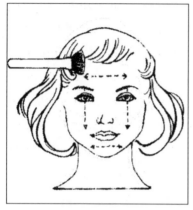

Apply Powder over Foundation

Go lightly on the powder. You can buy this in a cake form or loose. Loose is better because it spreads easily and is lighter than cake powder. To use: Dip powder brush in loose powder; tap off excess. Apply across forehead then down over each eye and cheek, and over chin area and along jawbone (as shown).

Beauty Step # 2: Smiling Eyes—The Windows to the Soul

Your next step is pretty eyes—and it's not only about makeup. The eyes have been called "the windows to the soul." I know mine always were for my parents, especially my mother. Several years ago when I was home for a visit, my mother knew instantly that something was bothering me. And she was right. It was a low period, a time when I just wasn't feeling all that great about my life.

I hadn't been home for more than two hours before my mother began ask-ing me how things were going. Knowing it's impossible to disguise my emo-tions when it comes to my mother's keen sense of intuition, I remarked, "Mom, you can always read me so well," and then asked her, "How do mothers know these things?"

"Your eyes," she replied, simply. "Your eyes don't have their usual sparkle."

My mother then took down a particular family photo album from the shelf where about a dozen sat. She flipped through the album to the different times of family life. "Look how happy you were during this time," she said. Flipping to yet another section, she remarked, "And look at these. This was during the time we moved and you left many good friends behind. You're smiling, but look at the sadness, the duress in your eyes. As I recall, this was a rough time for you. Now, look at this page," she said, yet again pointing to a series of photos. The new set she pointed out had been taken one afternoon after I had spent the entire morning horseback riding with my new friends from my new school. Smiling at me as she does in her usual loving way, she said softly, "I believe this renewed sparkle held the names Renee and Lindy!"

My mother was right. As I looked at the photos, I remembered my two new best friends and how fun that year was because the three of us were such good friends. Sure enough, my eyes looked happy, lighthearted and content. Happy eyes are vibrant eyes: What are yours saying? Vibrant eyes are beautiful eyes. Beautiful eyes are striking, appealing. Eyes that sparkle with warmth say that a person is happy, healthy. No makeup can create this kind of beauty—nor can any compensate for its being missing.

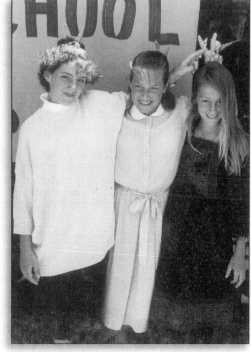

New best friends

As you read in unit 1, being happy is within *your* power, not that of others—though we sometimes think it is. It's important to make the decision to be a happy person. Too often, teens think that being happy is a result of what is happening in their lives. When things go the way we want them to, life is certainly more pleasant. But true happiness is more than that—it's a *decision* we each must make consciously, an *attitude* we each have to adopt. I know teens who, despite challenges they have to overcome, approach life with optimism—and with the intention to make their lives *all* that they can be, *all* they dream they will be.

There is no question that happiness and contentment play a role in dressing up our eyes. But in addition to these essentials, eye makeup that is skillfully and artfully applied can enhance and flatter the appearance of your eyes. Of course, you may not always want to wear eye makeup (especially to school every day), but if and when you do, here are ways to adorn your eyes.

Beauty Step # 3: Outlining Your Assets—Applying Eyeliner

Professional makeup artists think of your face as having "three eyes." Your own two, of course, and then their goal is to create the illusion that whatever the size of your eyes, that identical size of space is what they wish to create between them. This is their guideline for how far apart the eyes should "look" to others, a look that can be achieved by skillfully applying your eye makeup.

When you think of eye makeup, is mascara the first thing that comes to mind? While mascara certainly adds drama to the eyes, eyeliner is actually its most dramatic window dressing. Eyeliner gives the eye its real distinction. Whether you have round eyes or almond-shaped eyes, eyeliner makes your eyes look brighter, can change their shape and can also make your eyelashes look thicker [as you can see by comparing the two illustrations on the next page].

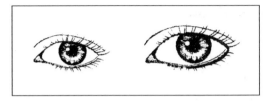 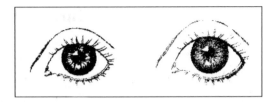

As a rule, you'll apply your eyeliner before applying any other eye makeup. Put it on before your eye shadow because it doesn't go on smoothly over eye shadow. Plus there's the advantage of being able to blend it to soften the way it looks if you apply your eye shadow over it. And, eyeliner goes on before your mascara so that it won't smear your mascara while you work on getting it in place.

Eyeliners and Eye Pencils

You can buy eyeliner in pencil, liquid or powder form. Which form of liner you choose is a matter of preference, but I like a pencil that is creamy enough not to pull the tissue around my eyes. When I use an eye pencil made of oil and wax, I can smudge the lines so they look natural and soft. However, if you have eyelashes that are really thin, a penciled line will be too thick for you to wear and you'll want to use a liquid instead. A word of caution: Pencils do have their problems. Because they're made out of wax, the color may run if you're out in very hot weather, and the pencil itself will melt if you leave it where it's too warm. It's not a good idea to carry it in your purse if you spend a lot of time outdoors. If you do take the eyeliner pencil to school, you might want to leave it in your locker.

Liquid eyeliner that is applied with a brush stays on very well, but it is not nearly as easy to apply as the pencil liner, which is why it isn't my choice in an eyeliner. Smudging can, however, be achieved by using a water-dampened cotton swab, brushing or dabbing to soften the overall look.

Tips for Using Eyeliner

- Because eyeliner is used to define the shape of your eyes, know what shape you're going for before you begin.
- For a very fine line, freshly sharpen your eyeliner pencil before each use.
- Draw a thin line as near to the base of your lashes as possible.
- If your pencil is too dry or hard, waving it in front of the heat from your blow-dryer for a couple of seconds should help make it creamier.
- If you apply color between all your lashes they'll look fuller.
- Be gentle with the delicate area around your eyes; avoid pulling on your skin.
- To blend your eyeliner so that you give yourself a soft appearance that looks natural, work the edges with a clean under-eye brush or an eye sponge.
- You always want your eyes to look natural, so you only want the barest hint of a line.
- Sometimes the brush might spread the liner more than you'd like. If this should happen you can use the sponge to remove any excess liner.

Beauty Step # 4: Shading with Eye Shadow

Eye shadows enhance the color and the shape of your eyes, and can make your eyes look larger, more dramatic and more expressive [as you can see in the illustrations below].

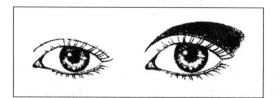 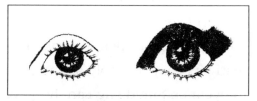

It's always best to buy it in fairly neutral colors, ones that flatter the color of your own eyes. In my freshman year in high school, all of my friends and I had to learn what colors really matched our individual coloring. My friend Lisa had yellow-green eyes and when she wore warm, yellow-green shades high-lighted with champagne shades, she looked great! But let her try wearing any-thing blue-green and it made her eyes look like they belonged on a clown. Remember, you're looking either for shades similar to your own eye coloring, or shades that complement rather than clash with it. The overall effect of eye shadow should be subtle, not bold.

Different Forms and Different Formulas

Not only does eye shadow come in different colors, it also comes in differ-ent forms—creams, crayons and pressed powders. There are even pressed powders that are molded into fat crayons. Here's the scoop:

- **Powders.** The most popular eye shadows are powdered. These are easiest to control when you are trying to smooth the color evenly over your eyelid. You can test your shadow by rubbing a little between your fingers (you want a powder that feels silky and not grainy or chalky). You're going to apply it with a brush or an eye sponge—using the eye sponge for blending heavier coverage and the brush for a lighter, very subtle look.

- **Creams.** Creams aren't the best form of eye shadow to use if you have oily skin because the color tends to slip off and build up in the creases of your eyelids. Creams can also be hard to apply and blend evenly. If you use one, dot it onto your eyelid using the tip of your finger, the tip of the eye wand or a clean under-eye brush. Then blend it in with a dry eye-shadow brush. This way, you can get the color to go on more pre-cisely before you blend it in.

- **Crayons.** Whether using a creamy eye crayon or a powdered one, you apply crayon coloring by drawing the color directly on your eyelids. It's best to blend the shadow with a clean, dry eye shadow brush or a stiffer contour brush. Powdered eye crayons blend really well and are easy to smooth into place on your eyelids. You have to press down harder when you use creamy eye crayons, so, again, be careful. Too much pulling and pressing can stretch the delicate skin around the eyes.

Tips for Getting Eye Shadow Perfectly in Place

It takes some practice, but you *can* get your eye shadow on evenly and learn to control it as you blend it into place. Here are some tips for how to master this skill:

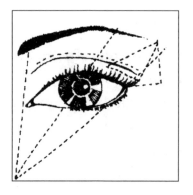

- Create a boundary to guide you in where to apply the eye shadow by picturing an imaginary line going from the outside corner of your eye to the outside tip of your eyebrow [as shown in the illustration].
- Keep your eyes open and look in the mirror while you're blending in the colors of your shadow (a magnifying mirror is best if you have one) so you can adjust the shape and check your boundaries.
- Start just above the crease in your eyelid, blending the color into the crease a little so that it will look natural.
- Use upward and outward strokes when you blend, going from the eyelid to the eyebrow. Your goal is to blend until the intensity of the color is just right and all the edges look smooth and natural.
- Make sure the shadow is placed high enough, because if it's too low or too close to the crease, your eyes will look like they are sunken in. (Also be careful not to place the shadow too low on the outside corner of your eye—it will make your eye look droopy.)

- To soften any color of shadow, use a light-brown or taupe powder, and a big soft brush and blend over the entire area where the color is too strong.

Beauty Step # 5:
The Magic Wand — Applying Mascara

The trick to having longer lashes that look thicker, fuller and darker is to use mascara. While you may choose to wear only mascara, if you're wearing mascara with other eye makeup, such as eyeliner and eyeshadow, you'll want to apply the mascara last.

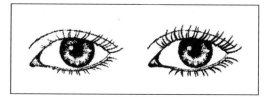 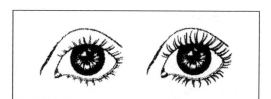

Cream, Cake or Liquid

Mascara comes in three forms: cream, cake and liquid. I don't recommend cake mascara because it runs easily from just the normal tearing of your eyes. Creams, which come in little tubes and need to be applied with a separate little brush, are much harder to get on your lashes evenly, so you can end up with a real mess trying. It's no wonder that liquids are the most popular—they are the most practical and easy to apply.

Liquid mascaras come in a tube with a wand inside, which is the brush you use to apply them. The little brush helps you separate your eyelashes at the same time you stroke on your mascara, so your lashes look longer and thicker. Some of the liquids even have added rayon or nylon fibers that stick to your eyelashes and make them look thicker—these are called lash builders. (You should never use a lash builder if your eyes are sensitive or you wear contacts, because the little fibers can irritate your eyes.)

You can buy liquid mascara in water-resistant and waterproof formulas, as well as the regular formulas. Regular mascara can streak or run if my eyes water for whatever reason, so I prefer to go with water-resistant mascara. It doesn't streak—not even when I work up a sweat during my aerobics class. The only time I use waterproof mascara is when I'm going swimming. It tends to make eyelashes really stiff, and you have to have a special makeup remover to get it off.

The Art of Applying Mascara: 6 Easy Steps

Step 1: When you take the wand out of the tube, make certain you get enough mascara on it—without getting any clumps on the wand. You may have to dip the wand in and out of the tube a few times to dispense the liquid over it evenly.

Step 2: Look in a mirror, tip your head back a little and gently stroke the mascara on your lashes with the little wand, lightly brushing all the lashes.

Step 3: Cover your lashes from the base to the tips by twirling the mascara

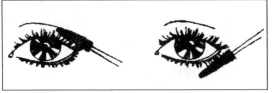

wand up and out over them. And here's a trick I learned from a makeup professional: Curl the lash with the makeup wand as you are waiting for the mascara to set. Just after applying the mascara, hold the wand at the base of the lash, and then slowly roll the wand up over the lash. This technique holds the curl longer, and is not as hard on your lashes as an eyelash curler. I'm not really fond of eyelash curlers, because I think they can hurt, I end up with watering eyes, and, in the process, I usually manage to lose an eyelash or two!

Step 4: If you choose to apply mascara to your lower lashes, lean your head slightly forward and twirl the wand down and out over the lashes.

Step 5: You'll always want to apply two coats, so repeat the above steps.

Step 6: Once both coats of your mascara are on, comb your lashes with a lash or brow brush to remove any clumps of mascara and to separate your lashes so they look longer.

Removing Mascara

Remove your mascara each evening when you wash your face, using either facial soap and water or eye-makeup remover. Gently remove with a cotton ball. Never use baby oil to remove mascara. Baby oil leaves a film of oil on your skin and clogs your pores. There are tons of products on the market to remove mascara; the best one is found in your school's theatrical room where the "movie stars" hang out: Abolene. It's a heavy-duty, tried-and-true cold cream, similar to the old-fashioned cold cream your grandmother used, and it's a great mascara remover, as well. After you've cleaned off the makeup, cleanse your face as usual.

Beauty Step # 6: Selecting the Right Frame—Your Eyebrows

The most beautiful masterpiece of art looks even more striking when it's set in the right frame. Eyebrows frame your eyes and your face. My friend, Janelle Paquette, has very pretty deep-green eyes that everyone admired—until last year when she all but tweezed her eyebrows bald and drew on lines to replace them. The problem was that the lines she drew on appeared totally unnatural. The result was that she looked clownish. The natural beauty in her sparkling green eyes was totally lost when offset by those eyebrows! The right frame for beautiful eyes looks balanced and even. Here's how to tell: Place a pencil from your nose and make a diagonal line directly to the middle of the eye. This point should be the highest place, the place where the eyebrow should arch.

It's "Tweeze-ee" to Have Great Eyebrows!

To achieve a balanced, even, lifted look for your eyebrows, you may have to pluck them into shape by using tweezers to remove stray hairs from the ends of them and from under the arch of your brow. Be careful not to pluck too much—eyebrows don't always grow back quickly, nor do they always grow back the same way there were. There's the possibility you could end up with a permanent mistake on your hands—or, more correctly, on your brows. To help avoid plucking hairs that you don't need to remove, first groom your eyebrows:

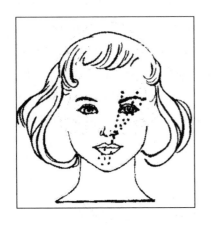

Step 1: Use a toothbrush or a brow brush to brush them straight up and down.

Step 2: Use cuticle scissors to snip off uneven points of hair.

Step 3: Brush the brow upward and outward to define the natural line.

If you've done this and your eyebrows still look like they need to be plucked, before doing so, cover the hairs you plan to tweeze out with concealer or foundation to see what your eyebrows will look like when they're gone. If you're okay with the way they will look, then you are ready to tweeze:

Step 4: Use your tweezers to grasp and pluck out unwanted hairs.

Step 5: Tweeze under your brow to form an arch.

You can soothe the sting of tweezing by rubbing the area with an ice cube.

Forming Great Eyebrows Using an Eyebrow Pencil

Plucking, along with using an eyebrow brush, may be all you ever need to do to have flattering, well-shaped eyebrows. But if you find that there are spots that you need to fill in where your eyebrows are too short, too thin, uneven or bare, you can use an eyebrow pencil and brush to get the look you want. Here are some tips:

- To pencil your brows, feather the color on in short, quick strokes.
- Don't ever just draw your eyebrows on; harsh lines look anything but natural!
- Once your lines are applied, use your lash/brow brush to brush your eyebrows up and out.
- For eyebrows that won't stay in place when you shape them, a little Vaseline and your brow brush can be just the trick. You can also brush them into shape with a toothbrush sprayed with a little hairspray.

Healthy Eyes: How to Avoid Allergic Reactions to Eye Makeup

Eye makeup, particularly mascara, is a good breeding ground for bacteria. Using a contaminated mascara wand or eyeliner pencil or eye shadow brush can give you an eye infection that looks awful and feels worse. A good rule is to toss any products that are older than six months.

If your eyes itch and turn red, look for hypoallergenic products. If switching to hypoallergenic products doesn't eliminate redness, or if you suspect that you have developed an infection, see a doctor.

Beauty Step # 7:
Go for the Glow—Brushing on Blush

A beautiful face has the healthy glow of color. Sometimes blush is used to enhance or create this glow. But again, makeup should look natural. Never is this more true than with blush. Remember that its role is to add a hint of color—and not to make you look like a clown! Skillfully applied, blush can actually change the appearance of the size of your face! For example:

- A narrow face can look wider if you start the blush at the outer corner of your eye and then blend the color straight back to your hairline at the center of your ear.
- A wide face can look slimmer by slightly blending your blush upward more toward the hairline just above each ear and then bringing it just a little bit lower than your nose at the other end.

Blush comes in different shades and not every shade looks good on everyone. For example, if you have dark skin, peach or brown shades of blush will be best for you. Pink shades have a subtle blue undertone that just won't work for your coloring—but they can work well with lighter skin. Shop around and try out different colors until you find the right one for you. Makeup consultants in department stores are a good source of advice on which blush is best for you.

Applying Blush

There are several different kinds of blush, including creams, powders, gels, liquids and mousses. One major difference between powders and all the other blushes is that you apply the powders with a blush brush, and the other forms with your fingertips. I wouldn't recommend gels or cheek tints because they dry fast and they're more apt to stain your cheeks and hands. As you can imagine, mistakes are a lot harder to correct with them. Mousses are a light, sheer foam that comes in aerosol cans. Unfortunately, mousse tends to run, so it can be fairly hard to get in place, especially in warm weather and when you perspire. If you decide to use a liquid or a cream blush, place three or four dots of the blush along the cheekbone with your middle fingertip. Then, gently smooth and feather the color with your ring and middle fingers until it blends in completely so that no edges show. My personal favorite is powdered blush, because I find it easy to blend to subtle shades that look natural. A large soft brush works best to spread the color evenly.

The secret to applying blush so that it flatters your face and looks natural is in how much you put on and where you place it. Here are some suggestions:

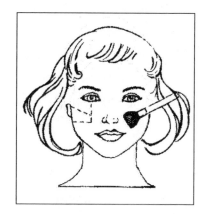

- As you apply blush, you need to be looking straight into the mirror. There's a tendency to turn your head to the side as you apply it. You want to see how it adds balance and contours to your face!
- Start your blush right under the outer edge of the iris of your eye. You can also place two fingers next to your nose to find this spot, and then start on the outside of those two fingers.
- From this point, blend the color out to the hairline at the tip of your ear.
- You'll want to have most of the color on the edge or top of the bone, which should be about at the outer corner of your eye.
- Feather slightly downward strokes within the hollow of your cheek, into a teardrop shape.
- Don't spread the color in the round area under your eye.

- Avoid going as high as your temple.
- Use a slightly stiff contour brush to blend all the edges so no line can be seen where your blush starts and ends.

Beauty Step #8: Smile with Style

A beautiful mouth begins with a great smile. A winning smile just might be your best beauty asset! Best of all, it's free, it's yours alone—and it never goes out of style! A smile says you are open, friendly, approachable. Let's say that a friend showed you each of the pictures on the next page, and said, "This is another friend of mine. Do you mind if she comes along with us on Friday to the mall window shopping?" Looking at each of the photos, which one would you feel more comfortable having along? I've tried this exercise many times. Most everyone said they would be more likely to enjoy the company of the girl (me) in the second photo, the Jennifer who is smiling. The point is, don't forget that your smile is one of your greatest beauty assets.

A Reason to Smile: Great Teeth

Along with having genuine happiness and kindness to convey, the biggest part of the beauty of a smile comes from having healthy, clean and well-cared-for teeth. This means brushing your teeth in the morning and before you go to bed at night, and flossing your teeth. It also means getting regular dental check-ups in prevention of gum disease and cavities. In addition, good dental care means eating the right foods and drinking milk every day so that you have the calcium and vitamins you need to keep your teeth strong. And it means—for many teens—the extra care and patience of wearing braces. When I was in the ninth grade, there were only eight kids in my class who didn't have braces. It's

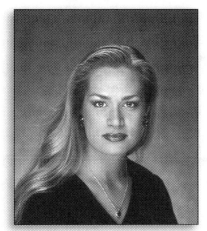

This girl . . .

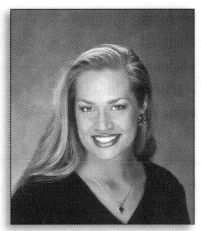

or this girl?

good news and bad news. At a time when you want to look great, chances are you have a mouth of metal! If you do wear braces, be patient. I wore braces, and it was a pain. The good news is great news: The result is that I now have straight teeth. (Of course, today, there are alternatives to metal braces; white-plastic braces are also used. I sure wish they had been available when I was a teen!)

Once you decide to share your smile and care for your teeth, you're ready for another Cinderella measure: lipstick!

Beauty Step # 9: The Perfect Paint—Lipstick

Remember when you were just a little girl and wearing your mother's lipstick was just the biggest-girl thing to do? I remember watching my mother apply her lipstick as she was getting dressed to go somewhere and being so enamored with the idea that one day I would actually be allowed to wear lipstick. Lipstick was like a rite of passage. Perhaps it will always be this way. When I was in the sixth grade, the biggest arguments I got into with my father were never over how I was spending my allowance or even about how my messy I was allowed to keep my room. It was about when I would finally be old enough to wear lipstick. I think his idea was that it should be when I entered high school. My mother was more cool about this. It was obvious to her that it was only natural that every girl in sixth grade was dreaming about her first lipstick. Her very own lipstick. And so she bought me a little tube of clear lipgloss. It was perfect. I treasured that little container. It was a reminder of the joy that, one day, I would have the *real* thing—colored lips!

S.W.A.K. (Sealed with a Kiss): Coloring Your Lips

Lipstick should complement your natural coloring. (If your parents haven't yet given their approval for you to wear lipstick, you might ask them if they will consent to a clear lipgloss.) Just as in the chapter where you learned that each of us looks best in certain colors, the different shades of lipstick look different depending on your natural coloring. The color of lipstick that looks awesome on a brunette with olive skin or a girl with black hair and a darker complexion may not look as great on a fair blonde. Likewise, the color of lipstick that looks just stunning on a girl with blonde or sandy-brown hair and fair skin will make a girl with dark hair look washed out.

If you are uncertain or just beginning to look for colors that look best on you, experiment until you find the shade that works best with your coloring. Enlist the help of your friends, and, in addition to their advice, ask at the makeup counter in your local stores. Most big stores have makeup consultants who offer their services for free.

Lip Tips

Although you can get them in little palettes or pans with brushes, lip color usually comes in tubes, pencils or creams. Here are some lip tips:

- Cream lipsticks stay on longer because they have both extra pigment and extra wax.
- Lipgloss has a moist, shiny look because it has more oil in it, but it doesn't stay on as long.
- Frosted lipsticks look pearlized and sparkling. They create a really nice evening or high-glamour look.
- Look for a lipstick with vitamins A and E in it. They're great conditioners and emollients.
- Beeswax and carnauba wax are two of the natural waxes that are always nice to find in lipstick. Not only do they give lipstick a lovely texture, they also help it glide on smoothly.
- Always look for lipsticks with a sunscreen. This helps keep your lips from drying out and cracking.
- Lipliners (or lip pencils) help define the shape of your lips.

Here are some steps for how to apply your lip color so that it shapes and flatters your lips:

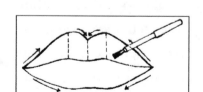 **Step 1:** Use a lip pencil or liner to define the shape you want, starting the line at the corner of your mouth, as shown. If you want to make your lips look smaller, use a pencil that is a little darker than your lipstick. You can also try applying the line just inside your natural lip line. If you want to make your lips look fuller, use a pencil or liner that is a little lighter than your lipstick. You can also apply your lipliner just outside your natural lip line. If your lips are unbalanced, apply the liner just outside

your natural lip line on the thin lip, and just inside your lip line on the full lip.

Step 2: Apply lipstick over the entire surface of your lips, smoothing it over one lip at a time.

Step 3: Press your lips together after you've applied the lipstick to spread the color evenly. Blot with a tissue to remove excess lipstick (this avoids the lipstick's looking too heavy, and prevents your wearing it on your teeth!).

"Face Value"

Although we wear makeup to add vibrancy and pizzazz, it should be more subtle than bold. Again, artful application is the key, and nothing can take the place of learning firsthand. Experiment until you get it down. I strongly suggest that you take advantage of getting your makeup done at a department store counter, or by a professional, at least once a year. (This is usually a free service, primarily because this is how the department stores "show off" the new products, and they're hoping that if you can see how to use them, and like them, you'll become a store customer. Sometimes, department stores will charge a minimal fee, like $5 or $10. Ask what their policy is before you schedule.) Not only is this enjoyable, but you'll find it's a real education. The important thing is that as you are sitting there having your makeup "done," rather than zoning out or getting caught up in observing the activities going on around you, pay close attention to the makeup and colors being used by the makeup professional, as well as to the techniques being used in the application of your makeup. And, by all means, speak up. Ask questions such as, "How did you achieve that look?" Or, "What color, brand or applicator are you using—and why? Can it be purchased? Where would I buy it? What does it cost?" Also, speak up about the results you are seeing. For example, "I love that color you're using, but I can't really see myself wearing it (to school) unless you can soften it. How would I do that?" Or, "I don't like that color on me. What other color would you suggest?" These are only a sampling of the many questions you should ask, but I think you get the idea. The goal is to educate yourself so you know what looks best on you and how to apply it correctly when you leave the store yourself—looking your best Cinderella!

And speaking of Cinderella, be sure to check out teen Carrie Hague [see below and colorplates 74–93] having her own makeup done by makeup artist Lois Pearl! Violà! Carrie, a Cinderella to be sure!

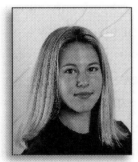

Before makeover

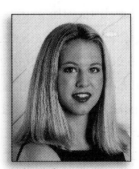

After makeover

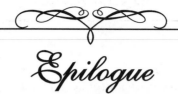

Epilogue

There you have it—suggestions and advice for looking and feeling great from your head to your toes, inside and outside. I hope this book has been a real health and beauty learning adventure for you, because writing it was for me! Of course, there's always more. If you're interested in getting further information, I've included a suggested reading section with great books you can turn to on each health, fitness and beauty topic we've covered, and more. As you'll note, I've listed them by chapter so you can easily find the ones that pertain to a subject you are interested in exploring.

I encourage you to use what you've learned and I support you in becoming your personal best. While you want to fit in, remember the goal is to dance to your own music, and shine and glimmer apart from the crowd—being good to your body and loving yourself for who you are. Enjoy being a part of the crowd, but don't be afraid to be an individual. You are you, and that's the point. It's your contribution to the world.

I've included my mailing address if you'd like to get in touch with me or let me know how this book has been helpful to you. And of course, I'd love to learn what other topics you would have liked to see covered. As always, take care, and don't forget to be a good friend—to others, and to yourself!

Taste Berries to You!

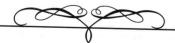

Suggested Reading

Chapter 1: If Only I Had Known in High School What I Know Now!

Coombs, H. S. *Teenage Survival Manual: How to Reach 20 in One Piece (And Enjoy Every Step of the Journey).* Laugunitas, Calif.: Discovery Books, 1993.

Feller, R. M. *Everything You Need to Know About Peer Pressure.* New York: Rosen Publishing Group, 1995.

Koyler, D. *Everything You Need to Know About Dating.* New York: Rosen Publishing Group, 1994.

Youngs, Jennifer Leigh and Bettie B. Youngs, *Taste Berries for Teens: Short Stories and Encouragement on Life, Love, Friendship and Tough Issues.* Deerfield Beach, Fla.: Health Communications, Inc., 1999.

———. *Taste Berries for Teens Journal: My Thoughts on Life, Love and Making a Difference.* Deerfield Beach, Fla.: Health Communications, Inc., 2000.

Chapter 2: The Radiance of *Inner* Beauty

Calderone-Stewart, Lisa-Marie. *Life Works and Faith Fits: True Stories for Teens.* Wynona, Minn.: St. Marys Press, 1999.

Honor Books Staff. *God's Little Instruction Book for Teens.* Tulsa, Okla.: Honor Books, 1998.

Johnson, Greg P. *If I Could Ask God One Question: Answers to Teens' Most Asked Questions.* Minneapolis, Minn.: Bethany House, 1998.

Peterson, Lorraine. *How to Get a Life. . . No Strings Attached: The Power of Grace in a Teen's Life.* Minneapolis, Minn.: Bethany House, 1997.

Meier, Paul D. and Jan Meier. *Happiness Is a Choice for Teens.* Nashville, Tenn.: Thomas Nelson, 1997.

Chapter 3: The Picture of Self-Esteem

Ignoffo, M. *Everything You Need to Know About Self-Confidence*. New York: Rosen Publishing Group, 1995.

Stewart, William. *Building Self-Esteem: How to Replace Self-Doubt with Confidence and Well-Being*. Philadelphia, Pa.: How To Books Ltd, 1998.

Youngs, Bettie B. *You and Self-Esteem: A Book for Young People*. Torrence, Calif.: Jalmar Press, 1996.

Youngs, Bettie B. and Jennifer Leigh Youngs. *Taste Berries for Teens Journal: My Thoughts on Life, Love and Making a Difference*. Deerfield Beach, Fla.: Health Communications, Inc., 2000.

Chapter 4: From "Me" to "You"

Fairview Press Editors. *How We Made Our World a Better Place: Kids and Teens Write on How They Changed Their Corner of the World*. Minneapolis, Minn.: Fairview Press, 1998.

Glassman, B. *Coping with Stepfamilies*. New York: Rosen Publishing Group, 1994.

Sidy, R. V. *Rebellion with Purpose: A Young Adult's Guide to the Improvement of Self and Society*. Sedona, Ariz.: SNS Press, 1993.

Youngs, Bettie B. and Jennifer Leigh Youngs. *Taste Berries for Teens Journal: My Thoughts on Life, Love and Making a Difference*. Deerfield Beach, Fla.: Health Communications, Inc., 2000.

Chapter 5: The Beauty of Purpose and Passion

Benson, Peter L., J. Galbraith and P. Espeland. *What Teens Need to Succeed: Proven, Practical Ways to Shape Your Own Future*. Minneapolis, Minn.: FreeSpirit Publishing, 1998.

Burnett, Patricia Hill. *True Colors, An Artist's Journey from Beauty Queen to Feminist.* Troy, Mich.: Momentum Books Ltd., 1995.

Covey, Sean. *The 7 Habits of Highly Effective Teens: The Ultimate Teenage Success Guide.* New York: Simon & Schuster, 1998.

Youngs, Jennifer. *Goal Setting Skills for Young Adults.* Second Edition Del Mar, Calif.: Learning Tools, l999.

Youngs, Bettie B. and Jennifer Leigh Youngs. *Taste Berries for Teens Journal: My Thoughts on Life, Love and Making a Difference.* Deerfield Beach, Fla.: Health Communications, Inc., 2000.

Chapter 6: Do You Like *Your* Body?

Moe, B. *Everything You Need to Know About PMS.* New York: Rosen Publishing Group, 1995.

Myerson, R. M. *How Your Heart Works.* Emeryville, Calif.: Ziff-Davis Press, 1994.

Pruitt, B. E., Ed.D., CHES, Kathy Teer Crumpler, M.P.H., and Deborah Prothrow-Stith, M.D. *Health Skills for Wellness.* Needham, Mass.: Prentice Hall, 1997.

Radiance: The Magazine for Large Women. P.O. Box 30246, Oakland, CA 94604. *www.radiancemagazine.com.*

Walker, Rebecca. *Adios Barbie: Young Women Write About Body Image and Identity.* Seattle, Wash.: Seal Press Feminist Pub., 1999.

Chapter 7: Fueling the Body Beautiful

Engel-Arieli, S. L. *How Your Body Works.* Emeryville, Calif.: Ziff-Davis Press, 1994.

Saltzer, C. A. *Looking Good, Eating Right: A Sensible Guide to Proper Nutrition and Weight Loss.* Brookfield, Conn.: Millbrook Press, 1991.

Saltzer, C. A. *The Nutrition-Fitness Link: How Diet Can Help Your Body and Mind.* Brookfield, Conn.: Millbrook Press, 1993.

Chapter 8: "You Are What You Eat": Making Smart Choices About Food

Jacobson, M. F., et al. *Safe Food: Eating Wisely in a Risky World.* Venice, Calif.: Living Planet Press, 1991.

Krizmanic, Judy. *A Teen's Guide to Going Vegetarian.* New York: Puffin, 1994.

Pruitt, B. E., et al. "Making Healthy Food Choices," In *Health Skills for Wellness.* Needham, Mass.: Prentice Hall, 1997.

Chapter 9: What You Should Know About Losing Weight

Ojeda, Linda. *Safe Dieting for Teens: Design Your Own Diet, Lose Weight Effectively, Feel Good About Yourself.* Alameda, Calif: Hunter House, 1992.

Sonder, B. *Eating Disorders: When Food Turns Against You.* New York: Franklin Watts, 1993.

Spies, K. B. *Everything You Need to Know About Diet Fads.* New York: Rosen Publishing Group, 1993.

Chapter 10: "Buffing Up" the Bod

Clayton, L. *Everything You Need to Know About Sports Injuries.* New York: Rosen Publishing Group, 1995.

Lang, Susan S., with Beth H. Marks. *Teens and Tobacco: A Fatal Attraction.* New York: Twenty-First Century Books, 1996.

Silverstein, H., V. Silverstein, and R. Silverstein. *Steroids: Big Muscles, Big Problems.* Hillside, N.J.: Enslow Publishers, 1992.

Simon, N. *Good Sports: Plain Talk About Health and Fitness for Teens.* New York: Harper & Row, 1990.

The Body Shop International, plc. *Mind, Body & Soul: The Shop Book of Wellbeing.* New York: A Bulfinch Press Book; Little, Brown and Company, 1998.

Chapter 11: Relaxing Your Body

Benson, Herbert, M.D., with M. Z. Klipper. *The Relaxation Response*. New York: Avon, 1990.

Davis, Martha, Eshelman, E. R., and M. McKay. *Relaxation and Stress Reduction*. Oakland, Calif.: New Harbinger Publishers, 1998.

Edelson, E. *Sleep*. New York: Chelsea House, 1992.

Licata, R. *Everything You Need to Know About Anger*. New York: Rosen Publishing Group, 1994.

Youngs, Jennifer Leigh. *A Stress Management Guide for Teens*. Second Edition. Del Mar, Calif.: Learning Tools, 1999.

Chapter 12: What Your Appearance Tells Others About You

Hilfiger, Tommy, and David M. Keeps. *All American: A Style Book*. New York: Universe Pub., 1997.

Seymour, Stephanie and Sarah Ferguson. *Beauty Secrets for Dummies*. Indianapolis, Ind.: IDG Books Worldwide, 1998.

Versace, Gianni. *The Art of Being You*. New York: Abbeville Press Inc., 1998.

Chapter 13: "Nothing to Wear"?

Gilbert, S. *Go for It: Get Organized*. New York: Morrow Books, 1991.

Miller, Nancy. *Clutterology: Getting Rid of Clutter and Getting Organized*. Ridgepath, Conn.: CPM Systems, 1998.

Smallin, Donna. *Unclutter Your Home: 7 Simple Steps, 700 Tips and Ideas* (Simplicity Series). Pownal, Vt.: Storey Books, 1999.

Chapter 14: What Looks Best on *Your* Body?

Hayman, Gale. *How Do I Look?* New York: Random House, 1996.

Nixon, Nancy and Palmer, P. *Looking Good: A Comprehensive Guide to Wardrobe Planning, Color and Personal Style Development*. Portland, Oreg.: Palmer Pletsch Pub., 1996.

Schwab, Ann. *Get Yourself Together: The Fashion Guide for Teens*. Lakewood, Colo.: Acropolis Books, Inc., 1987.

Chapter 15: What Colors Look Best on You?

Jackson, Carole. *Color Me Beautiful*. New York: Ballantine Books, 1984.

Spillane, Mary and Sherlock, C. *Color Me Beautiful's Looking Your Best: Color, Makeup & Style*. Lanham, Md.: Madison Books, 1995.

Chapter 16: It's the Little Things That Count: Accessories

Johnson Gross, Kim. *Accessories (Chic Simple)*. New York: Knopf, 1996.

Pullee, Caroline. *20th Century Jewelry*. North Brighton, Mass.: World Publications, 1999.

Reybold, L. *Everything You Need to Know About the Dangers of Tattooing and Body Piercing*. New York: Rosen Publishing Group, 1995.

Chapter 17: Shopping, Shopping, Shopping, Shopping, Shopping

Hoobler, Dorothy and T. Hoobler. *Vanity Rules: A History of American Fashion and Beauty*. New York: Twenty-First Century Books, 1999.

Klensch, Elsa. *Style*. New York: A Perigee Book, The Berkley Publishing Group, 1995.

Pooser, Doris. *Secrets of Style*. Menlo Park, Calif.: Tandy Brands Accessories, Inc., d.b.a. Always In Style, Crisp Publications, Inc., 1994.

Chapter 18: Scents-ible Advice: What You Should Know About Perfumes

Fischer-Rizzi, Susanne. *Complete Aromatherapy Handbook: Essential Oils for Radiant Health*. New York: Sterling Publishing, 1990.

Moran, Jan. *Fabulous Fragrances*. Beverly Hills, Calif.: Crescent House Publishing, 1994.

The Fragrance Foundation. *The Facts and Fun of Fragrance*. New York: Fragrance Foundation, 1992.

Chapter 19: Beautiful Skin

Barrick-Hickey, Beth. *1001 Beauty Solutions: The Ultimate One-Step Advisor for Your Everyday Beauty Problems*. Naperville, Ill.: Sourcebooks Trade, 1995.

Hammerslough, J. *Everything You Need to Know About Skin Care*. New York: Rosen Publishing Group, 1994.

Raichur, Pratima, with Marian Cohn. *Absolute Beauty: Radiant Skin & Inner Harmony Through the Ancient Secrets of Ayurveda*. New York: HarperCollins, 1999.

Chapter 20: Beautiful Hands and Nails

Cimaglia, Alice R. *Art and Science of Manicuring*. Albany, N.Y.: Milady Publishing Corporation, 1986.

Ferri, Elisa, Lisa, Kenny and Dana Epstein. *Style on Hand: Perfect Nail and Skin Care*. New York: Universe Publishing, 1998.

Manos, Fran. *Beautiful Hands & Nails Naturally*. New York: Avery Publishing Group, 1998.

Chapter 21: Fancy—and Comfortable—Feet

Mix, Godfrey. *The Salon Professional's Guide to Footcare*. New York: Milady Publishing Corporation, 1998.

Pritt, Donald and Morton Walker. *The Complete Foot Book: First Aid for Your Feet*. Garden City, N.Y.: Avery Publishing Group, 1996.

Tourles, Stephanie. *Natural Footcare: Herbal Treatments, Massage, and Exercise for Healthy Feet*. Pownal, Vt.: Storey Books, 1998.

Chapter 22: Simply *Beautiful* Hair

Barrick-Hickey, Beth. *500 Beauty Solutions: Expert Advice on Hair & Nail Care—What to Buy and How to Use It!* Naperville, Ill.: Sourcebooks Trade, 1993.

Caldwell, Margaret and Marjory Dressler. *Hair Designs: Fun and Fancy*. New York: Scholastic Trade, 1993.

Planet Dexter Editors. *The Hairy Book: The Truth About the Weirdness of Hair, Everybody's Hair—Untangled and Uncut*. New York: Penguin USA, 1996.

Pleasant Company Editors. *Beautiful Barrettes: Dazzling Designs to Create* (American Girls Collection Series: American Girl Library). Middleton, Wis.: Pleasant Company Publications, 1999.

Chapter 23: Dressing Up Your Face

Aucoin, Kevyn. *The Art of Makeup*. New York: HarperCollins, 1996.

Quant, Mary, David King, and Maureen Barrymore. *Ultimate Makeup & Beauty Book*. New York: DK Publishing, 1996.

Stacey, Sarah and Josephine Fairley. *The Beauty Bible*. New York: Overlook Press, 1997.

There is also a wealth of valuable health, fitness, beauty and fashion information online. If you own a computer, all you need is a modem and a phone—and, of course, your parents' permission. Fees for getting online vary; again, be sure you have your parents' permission.

Once you're up and online, search for informational Web pages by going to keywords such as beauty, fitness and health. You can also chat about subjects on Internet Relay Chats (IRCs) or newsgroups, such as "Health and Fitness," "Fashion," "Eating Disorders," and so on.

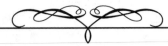

About the Author

Jennifer Leigh Youngs, twenty-five, is a speaker and workshop presenter for teens and parents nationwide. She is the coauthor of the bestseller *Taste Berries for Teens: Inspirational Short Stories and Encouragement on Life, Love, Friendship and Tough Issues* and *Taste Berries for Teens Journal: My Thoughts on Life, Love and Making a Difference;* and author of *A Stress-Management Guide for Teens* and *Goal-Setting Skills for Young Adults.*

Jennifer is a former Miss Teen California finalist and Rotary International Goodwill Ambassador and Exchange Scholar. She serves on a number of advisory boards for teens and is the International Youth Coordinator for Airline Ambassadors, an international organization affiliated with the United Nations that involves youth in programs worldwide to build cross-cultural friendships; escort orphans to new homes and children to hospitals for medical care; and deliver humanitarian aid to those in need around the world.

An avid sports enthusiast, Jennifer's hobbies include skiing, mountain biking, horse riding—both English and Western—and being with her friends. In high school, Jennifer was an editor for her school paper and lettered in varsity tennis, soccer and softball. Her peers voted her "Most Inspirational Player" three years in a row. Jennifer says that her overall goal in life is "to be happy and to make a difference. I'd like those who know me to feel enriched because I was in their lives. And I'd like those who meet me—even if for a brief moment—to feel they met a friend."

To contact Jennifer Leigh Youngs, write to:

Jennifer Leigh Youngs
Youngs, Youngs & Associates
Box 2588
Del Mar, CA 92014

Also from Jennifer Leigh Youngs and Bettie B. Youngs
The Taste Berries for Teens Series

The stories in these books will help you use the ups and downs of your bittersweet teen years to learn who you are and who you want to be.

The accounts from other teens about how they've dealt with issues will inspire you and give you hope.

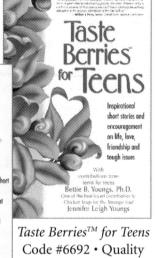

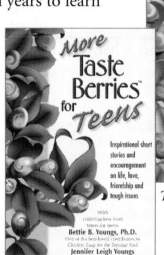

Taste Berries™ for Teens
Code #6692 • Quality
Paperback • $12.95

More Taste Berries™ for Teens
Code #813X • Quality Paperback • $12.95

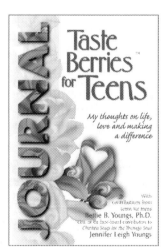

Taste Berries™ for Teens Journal
Code #7680 • Quality
Paperback • $12.95

An awesome journal that not only helps you focus on your innermost feelings, explore unlimited possibilities and describe your fondest dreams, but also-and even more important-to turn those possibilities and dreams into reality.

What's it all about?

Ever feel uncomfortable talking to your parents? Are there tough issues you're dealing with that you'd like to share with them, but don't know how? *Why Can't We Talk* is filled with writings from teens who share with heartfelt honesty the situations in their lives that they are unable to discuss with their parents. You'll read personal messages that'll help you realize that you're not alone.

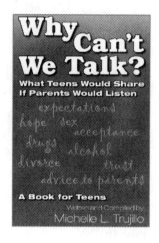

Why Can't We Talk
Code #7788 • Quality Paperback • $12.95

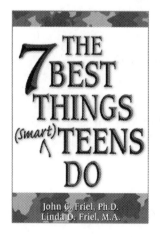

Still trying to figure out what this "life" thing is all about? Do you often wonder whether to listen to your heart or your head? This great new book will make you think, wonder, question and challenge yourself and show you seven of the most powerful tools you have to make your life a success and put it all perspective.

The 7 Best Things Smart Teens Do
Code #777X • Quality Paperback • $10.95